KW-483-804

HORIZON
AT THE FRONTIERS
OF MEDICINE

edited by

Simon Campbell-Jones

ARIEL BOOKS
BRITISH BROADCASTING CORPORATION

First published 1983
© BBC 1983

Published by the British Broadcasting Corporation
35 Marylebone High Street, London W1M 4AA

Typeset by Phoenix Photosetting, Chatham
Printed in England by Mackays of Chatham Ltd

Set in 10/11pt Linotron Ehrhardt

ISBN 0 563 17955 4

Contents

Introduction

Simon Campbell-Jones

A small group of medical scientists with a matching number of tele-vision producers were sitting around the lunch table. It was one of those semi-formal meetings at which representatives of the two professions try to come to terms with each other's problems. Friendly noises are made and accusations of trivialisation on the one hand and paranoia on the other are left behind. Nonetheless, one of the surgeons leaned forward and almost banged the table. 'When will you people realise,' he said, surprising everyone with his slightly raised voice, 'that medicine is not a science, it's an art.'

It seemed a fairly obvious remark on the face of it, not worth getting heated about, but it stuck in the mind. There is no doubt that medicine is an art. Intuition, an understanding of the individual patient and a heavy dose of psychology, if not downright thespianism, are all part of the doctor's skills. The profession can be criticised for not teaching enough of this to its students, but it's certainly not ignored in practice. Neither is it ignored in television programmes where not dissimilar 'human factors' can lift a medical story out of the clinical into the rivet-ing. So the implied criticism did not seem to be justified.

But what about the scientific frontiers of medicine – medical re-search? Is there art in the laboratory, in the pursuit of a bacterium or a virus, in the search for a specific antibiotic, in the trials to determine the metabolism of a new drug? Surely, in this area of medicine, strict scien-tific method is of paramount importance?

Perhaps not. Perhaps this is what the speaker was getting at. Medical research can be as creative, difficult, dubious and even as haphazard as any other scientific activity. But the 'art' is more specific than that. It is akin to the art of the detective. Evidence is gathered and carefully sifted. Facts are checked and re-checked. A case is built up that is as watertight as possible. Patients, or their case histories, can be pulled in for further questioning. Then fingers of accusation can be pointed at particular pathogens, and remedies can be put forward. But facts do not always fit neatly together. Intuitive leaps are required, some of which are wrong, some of which will always seem obvious with hindsight. Interpretation of the facts is always open to question.

Furthermore, false trails and red herrings abound. Time, effort and money are wasted. Manoeuvring and politicking often goes on between the leading characters, between laboratories, between institutions and governmental bodies, between differing commercial interests. Even the cultural backgrounds of the different investigators can change the way the research is approached. Nonetheless this is the 'art' that makes the stories interesting.

This book is a collection of such medical detective stories, based on Horizon *programmes and written by the producers concerned. It is a curious feature of the* Horizon *series that it is almost alone in taking a highly analytical, scientific approach and combining with it the element of suspense and surprise which is characteristic of detective stories.*

This is why the comment of the speaker at the lunch table riled. It was unfair. He would have been more accurate if he had said, 'Medicine is not just *a science, it's an art.' But even that is not good enough. He had fallen into the trap of separating science and art. It makes one sound dull and the other valueless. Those of us on the other side of the table were already well aware that scientific method is a tool. It is an indispensable tool which, if ignored, destroys the research and sometimes the researchers themselves. But it is their creative ability which is of value to their colleagues and to society as a whole. It is this combination of science and art which has over the years supplied a fund of fascinating stories for* Horizon.

The following pages will take the reader from Mill Hill to Peking, visiting on the way almost every part of the human body. They will show that the art of medicine is by no means an exact science, especially for those working at the frontiers of research. Anything can happen.

1 The Big IF . . . .

Vivienne King

January 1980. It was the start of a new decade – and with it, a new word burst into the headlines: interferon. Newspapers and TV programmes held out hope of a radically new treatment which could wipe out viruses. But more – it might cure cancer.

Interferon – IF to the scientists – is a new and special kind of drug. It's a natural substance made by the human body itself to fight infection. Though Interferon was new to the public, it had been discovered as long ago as 1957 by British Scientist Dr Alick Isaacs and a Swiss colleague, Jean Lindenmann. They were working at a time when antibiotics had revolutionised the treatment of bacterial infections such as TB or septicaemia; but they were not effective against viruses. Doctors used penicillin to treat the complications of diseases like measles or influenza, but for the viruses themselves there was neither treatment nor cure. The only hope was to prevent disease by vaccination: but vaccines were still in their infancy. Every year the headlines were filled with the frightening news of polio epidemics and deaths from influenza – or even from the vaccines themselves.

Working at the National Institute for Medical Research at Mill Hill in London, Isaacs was investigating a curious phenomenon called 'interference'. Doctors knew that it is rare for a patient to catch more than one virus at a time; the first infection somehow protects against others. But how? Isaacs set up an experiment to investigate interference. He injected hen's eggs with a flu virus. Inside the eggs, the chick cells retaliated by producing microscopic amounts of a protein. When Isaacs injected this protein into fresh, uninfected eggs, he found it made the new chick cells resistant to influenza – and other viruses. This magic substance was the key to interference. It was a most potent virus-blocker – and one of the most powerful biological agents ever found. He called it 'Interferon'.

Isaacs and his colleagues were filled with excitement. If they could tap the interferon from infected cells, they would have a

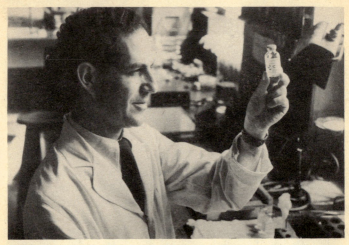

Dr Alick Isaacs

most powerful drug: something equivalent to the antibiotics, a magic bullet that could wipe out viruses. It was a major break-through for British Science, and the Medical Research Council set up a science committee to investigate. Interferon caught the imagination of the world of science – and of science fiction. Isaacs reacted with schoolboy delight when his new discovery featured in a Flash Gordon cartoon.

For the first few months, interferon research raced ahead. It turned out to be the first line of defence against all kinds of diseases. Within hours of infection, almost every cell in the body reacts by making interferon. The patient's blood serum contains high levels of it for about four days, until all the other defence mechanisms get going. Most living creatures make interferon: birds, mammals, reptiles and even plants react to infections in a similar way.

But the intitial euphoria was short-lived. Isaacs and his colleagues ran into two major hurdles. First, they were making their interferon in hen's eggs. So this was chick interferon – and it didn't work in humans. It seemed that interferon was species-specific: in other words, you need chick interferon for chick viruses, and human interferon for human viruses. So for trials on human patients, they had to find ways of making interferon from human cells. And that turned out to be very difficult.

Tapping the invisible elixir was another problem; for cells make interferon in only the tiniest amounts. It was like looking

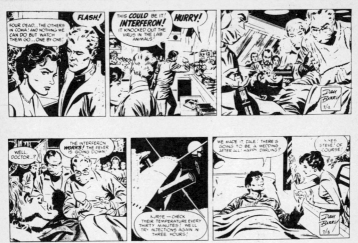

© 1983 King Features Syndicates.

for a needle in a chemical haystack. But most difficult of all was to purify it – and that problem took about twenty years to solve. Interferon is a very 'sticky' substance – other proteins cling to it. Scientists working with what passed for interferon were handling the crudest material: mostly impurities, very little interferon itself. Indeed, some of their early experiments were wrong: results were due to the impurities, not the interferon.

It was difficult to make, difficult to handle, and difficult to prove results. Gradually, scientists began to lose interest. They thought claims for interferon had been exaggerated. One American scientist even dubbed it 'misinterpreton'. And then Isaacs became ill. In 1964 he suffered an aneurism, a type of brain haemorrhage, which affected his speech. As a result, he became acutely manic-depressive.

His illness hardened attitudes to interferon. His widow, Susannah, recalls: 'One saw what one knows, really, that people are very frightened by mental illness, and frightened by mental illness in their own profession. And that made a lot of people very wary. I think some people thought it wasn't even true – that it had been just a wild idea, like the kind of wild idea that people get when they have a manic illness.' In 1967, Isaacs died. Few people still believed in interferon. Research went out of fashion as quickly as it came in. But a few disciples still remained, and it was largely through their persistence that the tide turned for interferon.

One of these was Barrie Jones. Working at Moorfields Eye Hospital, in London, he tested interferon on a type of herpes: herpes keratitis. This virus causes ulcers in the eye, and can lead to blindness. In the Sixties, it was incurable. After successful experiments on rabbits, Barrie Jones began trials on human patients. The interferon worked.

Next, years of apparently fruitless work paid off at the Cold Research Unit in Wiltshire. David Tyrrell and American scientist Tom Merigan pitted interferon against over a hundred viruses. They finally scored with Rhinovirus-4. Banner headlines proclaimed a victory for interferon against the Common Cold. But alas, Rhinovirus-4 was only one of thousands of cold viruses, and to cure it had cost £1000. For interferon was still scarce and difficult to make. Would it ever be more than a rich man's panacea?

While clinical trials were showing dramatic, if limited, success, in the laboratory the painstaking efforts of a few scientists were also beginning to pay off. By the late Sixties science had developed new techniques for probing the secrets of the living cell. Derek Burke, until recently Professor of Biological Sciences at Warwick University, was one of Isaacs' most loyal colleagues. 'Things really started to pick up because advances in other fields helped us to work on interferon – advances in biochemistry and in cell biology and genetics. So all of a sudden we had much better purification methods. All of a sudden we could investigate just how interferon did stop viruses from multiplying. All of a sudden we had different sorts of cells in which to study interferon production. All these things made it very much easier to really find out how interferon was made, what it was, and how it worked.'

Scientists had found that viruses are among the most primitive, yet insidious, forms of life: mere fragments of nucleic acid, the basic chemical from which all living things are built. They cannot even reproduce alone. To do so, they have to infect the cells of some other organism. Once lodged there, they use the genetic machinery in the nucleus of those cells to live and multiply.

The cells react by making interferon. This acts like a chemical alarm signal: molecules of interferon stream out of the dying cells to spread the news of invasion. They lock on to uninfected cells and induce them to make a new protein – antiviral protein – which prevents the invading virus from multiplying. This is the first stage of the interferon operation: meanwhile, it is alerting the rest of the body's defence mechanisms, and priming them for attack.

Injecting interferon is like injecting an alarm signal into a sleepy immune response: it stimulates the body to heal itself. Most other drugs are poisons: they kill both infected *and* healthy cells. Interferon boosts the body's own defences. But this was only the first of interferon's many secrets. A major surprise still lay in store.

Unable to obtain backing from disenchanted funding bodies, American scientist Ion Gresser had moved to Europe to continue his research on interferon. In his Paris laboratory, he made a chance discovery which was to change the fate of interferon. Gresser was using interferon to treat mice infected with a virus which caused cancer. The aim was to study its effects on the virus. But to his amazement he found it shrank the tumours.

Further investigation revealed that interferon has a dramatic effect on cancers. It slows down cell growth and reduces the size of tumours; and it also has the bizarre effect of making tumour cells look foreign. The body is primed to attack them exactly as if the tumour were a virus. So interferon's attack on cancer is two-pronged: it slows down cell-growth, and stimulates the production of killer cells to attack the tumour.

It was a totally unexpected bonus. The bogey of cancer looms large in everybody's fears – and the prospect of a new biological approach to treatment spurred on interferon research.

Gresser made one other major contribution that clinched the clinical potential of interferon. He found that it could be made in relatively large quantities from human blood cells. His work was taken up in Scandinavia. In Helsinki, Kari Cantell had an office next door to the Red Cross, headquarters of the Finnish blood transfusion service. This gave him an idea for the world's first interferon production line.

When a donor's blood is processed for transfusion, only the red blood cells are used. The rest usually ends up down the drain. But in each pint of blood are millions of white cells called leucocytes – potent producers of interferon, as Gresser had shown. Cantell rescued them from the sluice – brewed them up with a virus called Sendai – and turned them into interferon factories. It took many patient years to perfect the process; but by 1970, Finnish blood was supplying the world with interferon to try on human patients. Cantell's production-line opened up the first really fruitful lines of treatment in some previously hopeless diseases.

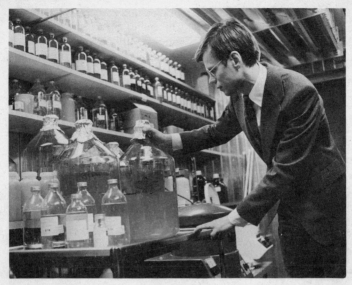

Professor Kari Cantell holds a bottle containing crude interferon. It takes about 400 blood donors to produce 23 litres of this crude material. Much purification and concentration are needed before it can be given to patients.

Trials with human cancer patients began in 1971, at the Karolinska Hospital in Stockholm. Hans Strander tested interferon on patients with a rare form of bone cancer – osteogenic sarcoma, a disease which strikes in adolescence. Doctors believe it may be triggered off by the sudden spurt in bone growth. At that time the only treatment was amputation; but this did not stop the spread of secondary cancers. Most patients did not survive for more than two years.

Strander was convinced that interferon worked. More than half the 43 patients treated are still alive. They have survived for over five years, without debilitating radiation treatment or chemotherapy. In fact, interferon opened up new ways of handling the disease. Caught early enough, there was no need for amputation; surgeons simply removed the tumours and replaced the diseased bone with grafts from healthy limbs. Furthermore, the interferon did not seem to produce the horrific side-effects associated with other cancer drugs.

But Strander's work was heavily criticised. Most scientific trials are conducted 'double-blind'. This means that only half the patients receive interferon. Doctors must not know which, so that results will not be biased by hope. Strander had merely compared the progress of his patients with case-histories from other hospitals. Doctors at the Karolinska now feel ethically bound to treat all their patients with interferon. They believe that without it, many would die, or suffer mutilating operations. But without the double-blind trials they can't really prove it.

While these results remain controversial, Strander has also done convincing work with another form of bone cancer called myeloma. In contrast to osteogenic sarcoma, this affects the old. His most impressive case was a man in his seventies who arrived at the Karolinska complaining that he couldn't put his hat on. The reason was a massive tumour on the back of his head. Four years previously, his wife had died from breast cancer in the same hospital. She had suffered badly from the effects of chemotherapy, and he was horrified when doctors put him on interferon.

But after three months of treatment, his tumour vanished. Apart from a slight fever with the first shot, he'd suffered no side-effects; his hair had not fallen out and he felt well. And he could wear his hat.

But Strander's most spectacular success has been with a viral disease of the very young, called laryngeal papilloma. Small, wart-like tumours grow in the throat. Though these are not malignant, they may well block the larynx so that the child chokes to death. Until now, the only treatment has been repeated operations – in the case of one young patient, as many as four hundred. As fast as surgeons remove the papillomas, they grow again. As a result of all this surgery, some children lose their voices. Strander put his patients on a course of interferon shots, given to them at home by their parents or the district nurse. He had one hundred per cent success. So far, only one child has permanently recovered. The rest rely on the weekly shots to keep the disease at bay. But most children grow out of it at puberty, so the treatment will not be for life. And there's a bonus – on interferon, they don't get colds.

While Strander pursued his cancer studies, Tom Merigan was also beginning clinical trials at Stanford University Medical Centre in California. He ran a promising trial with non-Hodgkins's lymphoma, a cancer of the lymph-glands. But he was also interested in the other great potential use of interferon – as an antiviral drug. After his brief excursion into the sneezing world of the Cold Research Unit, he turned his attention to other, more serious, chronic virus infections. Most patients eventually recover from a virus. But sometimes the body's immune response fails to overcome the infection, and the virus takes permanent hold. Such a disease is chronic hepatitis, a disease of the liver which can lead to death from cirrhosis or cancer. Until now, there has been no cure.

At first, results were inconclusive. Then Merigan tried combining interferon with another antiviral drug called Ara-A. And four of his patients were cured. The virus was knocked out – and blood tests showed that they had actually become immune to hepatitis. There was no possibility of a relapse.

The treatment did not work for all Merigan's patients, and the trial is continuing. But meanwhile he is experimenting on more exotic viruses, like rabies, and on common ones, like shingles. At Stanford, many patients have little resistance to infections because of drug treatment for cancer or transplant operations. These patients are especially vulnerable to common viruses like shingles or pneumonia. The hope is that interferon could improve their chances by cutting down the risk from secondary infections.

In England, a trial on similar lines is being carried out by Dr Phillip Gardner, who is using interferon to treat children with leukaemia. Modern drugs can keep the disease at bay – but by lowering their resistance to infection. The young patients may survive their leukaemia, but die from measles.

Gardner is conducting a double-blind trial on measles. It is not yet completed, but he tells a hopeful story. One young patient made such a dramatic recovery from a near-fatal attack that Gardner telephoned Kari Cantell in Helsinki to give him the news. Cantell supplies the material for the double blind trial in numbered phials. It was such an unusual story that Cantell broke with convention. He looked up the code, and found that the child *had* been treated with interferon.

By the end of the Seventies, the case for interferon was growing. But the evidence still amounted to little more than a few dozen anecdotes. No more than 150 patients in the world had been treated with it. And it doesn't work for everybody. Doctors still cannot predict with certainty which patients will respond to interferon – or even which diseases.

Hans Strander summarises: 'One could say that there is an effect of interferon on very many different tumours, but we don't know how strong the effect is as compared to treatments which are available already today. And there is also one other important point: that is that we have not been able yet to construct trials which are big enough to help us to decide how to give the interferon in an optimum way. I mean, maybe we should give five times more interferon, or we should give it, not every day, but once a week. It's very difficult to control all these factors in these initial studies.'

To answer all these questions would require massive international effort – and a huge investment. Until recently, most of the foot-slog had been done in the laboratories of Europe. But towards the end of the Seventies, a vigorous campaign was being fought in USA.

Leading the campaign was one of America's richest ladies, Dr Mathilde Krim. In 1970 she had prepared a report for Congress on the current state of cancer research – and helped get the US cancer programme off the ground. She had become convinced that the future lay in 'biologicals' – drugs which stimulate the body's own defence mechanisms, rather than poisoning both diseased and healthy cells. But the Americans had always been slow to accept interferon. Despite her connections and some influence in government circles, her campaign met with tough opposition.

'Whether the scepticism was founded or not is a matter of opinion,' says Krim. 'Perhaps in some cases one can say that it resulted from ignorance and lack of imagination, and lack of vision, rather than being well-founded. This is my opinion. I felt that at least ten years ago there was ample justification already for trying to produce human interferon and test it in man against a variety of diseases.'

Krim has enough private wealth to set up a small interferon factory of her own in Switzerland, supplied with blood cells by the Swiss Red Cross. She is a scientist herself, and director of interferon research at the Sloane-Kettering Memorial Institute in New York. Thus, she is able to organise academic research. But the drug companies she approached were not prepared to make long-term investment without proof that interferon would work. The only hope lay in Government agencies – but they were just as reluctant.

'Bureaucrats tend to be timid,' says Krim. 'They find it difficult to gamble with large amounts of money because they are accountable to the public. And altogether, the difficulty of the experiments, the reluctance of the industry to invest in this field, and the timidity of government agencies, have resulted in delaying by at least ten years the developments that were necessary.'

In 1978, something happened in America which changed the course of interferon history. Dr Jordan Gutterman of Houston, Texas, made bold claims for the success of interferon with breast cancer. Though only four patients had responded to the treatment, the story was much publicised. The American Cancer Society made an unprecedented offer of two million dollars to buy interferon for clinical trials. Patients lobbied Congress. The government-funded National Cancer Institute was forced to join in to the tune of a staggering eight million dollars. With increased pressure from Government, that sum continued to grow. Interferon fever had hit America.

But where could the Americans buy ten million dollars' worth? There wasn't that much in the world. Most of the trials conducted in the Seventies had used material made in Cantell's laboratory. The world depended almost entirely on Finnish blood for its supply of interferon. The method is expensive, and yields are low. Two million dollars' worth of interferon treats only 150 patients, and for only three months. Could Kari Cantell supply the proposed American trials? His answer was an emphatic 'No'.

'Well, we certainly cannot meet that demand. It seems to me that most pharmaceutical companies are waiting for more and more evidence of the clinical usefulness of interferon. But I don't understand how such additional evidence could be obtained, because there is not enough interferon available to do the clinical studies. So there is a vicious circle. And I think this vicious circle should be broken, and more interferon should be produced by the methods currently available.' But to supply all the cancer patients even in England with Cantell-type interferon would take a lot of blood-donors; there wouldn't be enough people in the world.

New methods of production were needed; and by the end of the Seventies, that race was on, with rich pickings promised for the winners. 'Interferon' had been a word restricted to academic circles and esoteric science journals. Now it featured daily in the financial press. At an international conference in New York in the autumn of 1979, scientists rubbed shoulders with men from Wall Street. Venture capital companies were set up virtually overnight. And all this at a time when scientific knowledge of interferon was very far from complete.

They didn't even know the chemistry of this magic molecule, for it had never been purified one hundred per cent. Doctors still had misgivings that its amazing effects could be due to impurities contaminating the mixture they were injecting into patients. For each shot contained as little as one per cent of pure interferon. And there was no evidence at all that interferon had ever 'cured' anybody. For all anyone knew, successful patients could be in a long, but temporary, remission. And there could be unimagined long-term side-effects.

Despite all these doubts, some drug companies decided to bite on the 'magic bullet'. They were taking an unprecedented risk, but hopes were high, and so were the financial stakes.

Front-runner in the race was a British company, Burroughs-Wellcome. By 1979 their pilot plant in Beckenham was already producing test samples of interferon by a revolutionary new method. In charge of the scheme were Dr Norman Finter and Dr Karl Fantes. Both had remained staunch believers in its potential when other interest dropped. Fortunately, they joined Burroughs-Wellcome in 1971 and put the company ahead with a bizarre method of production. Instead of using blood cells, they make their interferon in human cancer cells from the tumour of a little Nigerian girl called Namalva. The disease transformed her cells so that they continue to grow and multiply, though she has died. With this infinite supply of human cells, interferon production is continuous.

The major problem has been purification. They have to be certain that it's safe to treat cancer-patients with a drug that's made from cancer. Namalva suffered from a disease called Burkitt's lymphoma, known to be caused by Epstein-Barr virus. Burroughs-Wellcome had to guarantee that no dangerous fragments of the virus could leak into their interferon.

Karl Fantes devised an ingenious method. The details are highly secret – but Burroughs-Wellcome interferon has met the most stringent demands of British safety councils and America's Federal Drug Administration.

By early 1981 they had secured a slice of the American NCI's eight million dollar contract. They were supplying MRC-sponsored clinical trials in Britain, and research in universities at home and abroad. They had scaled up their pilot plant to commercial size and were marketing their technology to buyers in Japan.

But it was still a risky enterprise. Burroughs-Wellcome had made a massive investment. Even at 1980 prices, it would be at least five years before they recouped their losses. And what if some new, more efficient, and ultimately cheaper method of production should undercut them?

The challenge came from that new generation of biotechno-crats – the genetic engineers. Around the world, teams of scientists were engaged in a feverish race to set up a microbial production line for interferon. The aim: to isolate the human gene which codes for interferon, and switch it into the DNA of a bacterium. Switch on that gene – and the bacterium will make human interferon. Once such a strain has been successfully engineered, the bacteria can be farmed for ever – to produce an infinite supply of interferon, as cheap as penicillin.

Research was being carried out under a security net so tight that it would have done justice to a military operation. For it seemed there were golden stakes to be won. By the autumn of 1979, rumour ran rife that several American groups were near to success. Then in January 1980, an announcement was made by a European company called Biogen. Swiss scientist Charles Weissmann had succeeded in splicing the interferon gene into a bacterium – and making interferon. Weissmann's colleague, Harvard scientist Walter Gilbert, spoke boldly at a Boston press conference. 'The Eighties could be the decade which sees virus infections wiped out – and the opening up of new ways to control cancer.'

The news was received with cautious acclaim. There were a number of drawbacks. First, Weissmann's bacteria were producing miniscule amounts of interferon: only one molecule per cell of bacteria. Efficiency would have to be improved a million times to match the existing techniques. Secondly, how could they be sure that interferon produced in bacteria would work in the human body?

But though many problems were foreseen by the sceptics, everything turned out much easier than could ever have been expected. Within a year of Biogen's first breakthrough, several other groups, in America, Europe and Japan, had their own interferon-making bacteria, including a team led by Derek Burke at Warwick University. Weissmann had increased his yield by tens of thousands – and by spring 1981, bacterial interferon was going into patients. Though its effectiveness was still not proved, fortunes were being made in anticipation. When the Californian company Genentech went public in October 1980, the stock-market went mad. Two scientists who had originally invested $500 suddenly found themselves worth millions. Such was the commercial grip of the word 'interferon' on the public imagination.

Research which had taken so long to get off the ground was

now making dizzy progress. Elsewhere in the laboratory there were more breakthroughs: one problem to be cracked in 1980 was purification. British scientists David Secher and Derek Burke developed a technique for inducing mouse cells to make interferon antibody. These antibody molecules can be used to make a chemical sieve for separating out the interferon from an impure brew. Pass the mixture through a layer of antibody – and the interferon molecules will snap onto the antibody like iron-filings sticking to a magnet. Everything else slips through – only the pure interferon is left behind. Since the mouse cells can be grown ad infinitum, this antibody can be produced cheaply in limitless amounts. It means that interferon can be purified on a large scale.

By the end of 1980, what had seemed like a pipe-dream only two or three years previously was now being turned into reality: the possibility that pure human interferon could be manu-factured on a commercial scale. Meanwhile, in laboratories around the world, unsung heroes and heroines were pushing back the barriers to our understanding of interferon and how it works. By the beginning of the decade, it was already known that there were at least three different types of interferon: different body cells produce chemically different interferons which act in different ways.

Apart from the familiar leucocyte interferon, there is fibroblast interferon. It's made from solid tissue, muscle and skin. Most laboratories use human foreskins as raw material. Then there's a third type, called immune interferon, which has one very special property: mixed with either of the other two, it has an enhancing effect. The blend of interferons is at least ten times as effective as either one alone: a remarkable way of strengthening the action of interferon on both tumours and viruses.

These three interferon types have now been renamed: leucocyte interferon is α – interferon; fibroblast interferon is β – interferon; immune interferon is γ – interferon. By the end of 1980, scientists had discovered that there were even many differ-ent types of leucocyte interferon – at least eight, probably ten, and possibly even as many as sixteen. This variety could account for the fact that patients respond to interferon in such different ways.

The role of these types in fighting disease was also becoming clearer. It seemed that fibroblast interferon could be more effec-tive against solid tissue tumours like lung cancer; while leucocyte interferon might work better for bone or blood diseases. In virus infection, it emerged that interferon has a role in regulating the body's immune response: as well as switching it on, it also swithces it off. The latter is a crucial role, for without such a mechanism, we might turn into giant crystals of antibody, while reacting to infection.

Research into interferon was building up a clearer picture of how the body fights disease; and it was also contributing fundamental new knowledge to cell biology. Even if interferon fails to fulfil its hoped-for role as a panacea against viruses and cancer, it will have thrown fresh and important light on the workings of the living cell.

And what of its clinical potential? Extensive trials are needed on a world-wide basis, to discover which patients and which diseases will respond to which types of interferon; what dosage is required, and whether there may be long-term side-effects. There are no short-cuts to those answers; but two ingenious scientists have devised laboratory methods to prevent time being wasted.

In London, Joyce Taylor studies breast cancer by growing it in specially-bred mice. These mice are born with no immune response. They could not survive outside their sterile plastic tents in her laboratory, for they have no resistance to infection. Joyce is able to transplant tiny samples of human breast-cancer into these mice, for just as they cannot fight germs, so they cannot reject transplants. The mice are unaffected by the foreign cells, but the tumours grow well.

Once they are established, Joyce treats the mice with interferon. She has found it stops the tumours growing. Since the mice have no immune response, it cannot be their body defences which affect the cancer cells. The interferon must be acting directly on the tumours. To do such a trial on human patients would take years. Joyce has obtained her results in a few short months. It doesn't prove that interferon would cure the patients from whom the samples have been taken – but it does confirm that interferon has potential. As soon as more of the drug becomes available, breast cancer will be a strong candidate for clinical trials. In America, such studies have already begun.

In San Francisco, Lois Epstein has devised another laboratory technique for testing interferon – this time, on ovarian cancer. With cells drawn from patients' abdominal fluid, she can grow a tumour in a test-tube – in just three weeks; and that's how long it takes her to do an interferon trial.

In over seventy per cent of the samples she's tested, the

tumour shrinks. The next step will be to see if treatment that's effective in the test-tube is also effective in the patient. If so, it may soon be possible to predict whether a patient will respond to interferon by a simple laboratory test: vital at a time when the drug is still relatively scarce and expensive.

Much work remains to be done before interferon can meet the demands of an already clamouring public. It is, perhaps, unfortunate that its headline fame should have so outstripped its availability and proven worth. Patients treated successfully with interferon may well be on the drug for life – which means production must be vastly increased if it is ever to be used worldwide for everyday treatment. Even the Shah of Iran with all his wealth was unable to buy time with interferon – it simply wasn't available.

In Britain, we have already seen the dangers of too much publicity, too soon. In 1980, two teenage boys were treated in Glasgow with interferon bought from a manufacturer in Denmark. Despite apparent improvement in the first few weeks, both died. Apart from the private grief of families whose hopes were dashed, public failure of an untried drug could be its death-knell – there was a danger that drug companies might once again lose faith and cut their investment.

So the public must be patient. As Hans Strander said at the end of 1979, 'At the moment, it's not a wonder drug against all diseases. It's a substance which has been shown to have an effect on some virus diseases, and some tumour diseases. And that's it. And now comes a time of hard work, for we have to show how good the effect really is, and how it compares with other treatments.'

The lightning advances of 1980 have made that work possible. Massive clinical trials have already begun in Britain and America. Almost twenty years after Alick Isaacs' death, his faith in interferon is being put to the test. Let's hope that, one day, his 'IF' may become a certainty.

The excitement about interferon has subsided. It hasn't gone away; scientists are still hard at work. But what went wrong? Why did it not live up to its initial promise? Apart from the fact that publicity pushed expectations beyond any reasonable hope of fulfilment, there is something missing. The facts don't quite add up and there is a gap in the chain of events. Interferon only rings the alarm bells in the body's defence system, it doesn't actually attack the invaders. It encourages uninfected cells to wake up to the danger of a virus and it makes cancer cells visible, but that's it. Other mechanisms do the fighting. The connection between the two defence systems is not clearly understood. Injecting interferon is like adding extra alarm bells – it might work but there's no real reason why it should if the main defence system is already defective, which is the case with a patient who is really ill.

More detective work is needed and will, eventually, produce more answers. Then the excitement may rise again, but probably never as much as over another illness which is scarcely an illness at all.

An unbelievable amount of literature is published on the business of slimming. Only rarely is fatness a serious medical condition; and yet the interest in ectomorphs and endomorphs, 'fattypuffs and thinifers', sylphs and weightwatchers, never wanes. Maybe it's because no one has come up with a satisfactory explanation for the differences – until recently. One Horizon team found itself smack in the middle of the action as the process of discovery was going on.

2 The Fat in the Fire

Martin Freeth

For years folklore and medical orthodoxy have combined to make fat men and women feel guilty because they are fat. 'You eat too much,' they are told again and again. It is hard enough for a fat person to live with the prejudice of friends, who are quite sure he must be secretly eating between meals. But when even his doctor smiles knowingly and refuses to believe the most vigorous denials of gluttony, he begins to feel that somehow, despite appearances, he must be consuming more than his leaner fellows.

Some researchers, in particular Dr Derek Millar at Queen Elizabeth College, London, have insisted for years that the amount of energy people can burn off as heat is just as important in determining body weight as the amount of energy taken in as food. When the *Horizon* team was starting research into the causes of obesity, it was luckily just at the time when important discoveries were being made about the mechanisms involved in this burning up of surplus food.

When they published their findings the (mainly British) scientists involved quite literally put the fat in the fire. The research we reported, though it is still controversial, is helping to overturn a number of preconceptions about obesity.

Early in our researches, Dr John Garrow at the Northwick Park Hospital told us about the case of the famous William Campbell. When he died aged 22 he was 340 Kg. If his lean body mass was 90 Kg. that means he was carrying 250 Kg. of fat. That is equivalent to 1,750,000 calories. It sounds a great deal, but to accumulate this amount of fat by simple overeating, he would only have had to eat 218 excess calories a day. People need about 3000 calories a day, so 218 represents only a seven per cent imbalance of input over output.

Normally, metabolic rate (that is the rate at which people burn up food and/or stored body fuel) differs from individual to individual by much more than seven per cent. Many people can eat

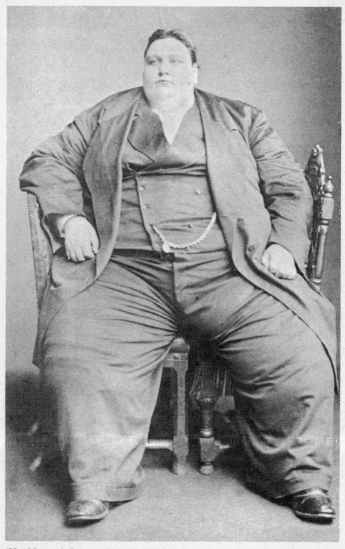

'Her Majesty's Largest Subject', William Campbell, weighed 340 Kg when he died in 1878 – but his intake of food may have been no more than average.

much more than they need and stay slim. So there must be a very fine control system which keeps the energy equation in balance over long periods, and prevents the majority of us sharing Campbell's fate.

Until recently most scientists, like most members of the public, have assumed that the fine control system must work principally on the input side, setting the level of our appetite and so controlling what we eat. Try as they might, the scientists could not discover such a fine-control system for intake.

The idea that fat people eat more than thin is so deeply ingrained that, even if we see him take only a single mouthful, we think an overweight person looks greedy. The truth can only be established by careful scientific measurements of intake and of output. Dr Philip James and his colleagues at the Dunn Clinical Nutrition Centre in Cambridge measure the calorific value of every ounce of food their patients consume. And for up to two months at a time the patients are honour-bound not to visit the local pub, and not to accept sweets from strangers – special tests being devised to ensure that they comply!

More importantly, Philip James confines patients for hours at a time to a 'room-calorimeter', where their resting metabolic rates are measured. The researchers then watch how metabolic rate is affected by taking exercise and by eating meals. Dr James also confines thin people to the calorimeter in the same way.

What is the difference between the two groups? You might think it would lie in the amount of exercise fat and thin people take, but this is not so. You can lose a lot of weight by sweating when you take exercise, but in fact it's soon replaced when you next take a drink. Whatever the health benefits of taking exercise, it is a very slow way to lose *fat*. You would have to walk briskly for an *extra* two hours a day to lose the fat equivalent of one piece of cake. Measurements in the calorimeter show that a far larger proportion of food energy is consumed just by sitting still and getting on with one's normal body chemistry. And it is somewhere in these routine metabolic processes that the difference between fat and thin people is to be found.

This is a metabolic 'difference' rather than a 'defect'. First of all, and again contrary to popular myth, it is only gross overweight that is correlated with ill-health. It is certainly unfashionable in our culture to be a bit overweight, so that can lead to much unhappiness – but according to Philip James at least, to carry a few extra pounds is no guarantee of illness or low life-expectancy. And in less extravagant and more deprived societies those who burn off food energy rapidly do less well. From an evolutionary point of view, what animals and humans need is a flexible form of control: to be able to store energy in hard times, but to burn off surplus food at a time of plenty. So when long-term overeating causes long-term increases in a person's metabolic rate, that is the process scientists are looking for. They call it 'diet-induced thermogenesis'.

Derek Millar proved over ten years ago that you could over-feed both pigs and students for long periods and that some individuals would nonetheless stay lean. A more dramatic experiment was conducted at the University of Vermont in 1974 by Dr Etham Sims at the Vermont State prison. He persuaded prisoners to volunteer to eat 3000 extra calories a day on top of their normal prison food for six months. Again, some individuals stayed lean. How had they burnt up the surplus calories?

One problem for Dr James if he, also, found metabolic differences between fat and thin subjects, would be to demonstrate that the differences are the *cause* and not the effect of being fat or thin. So he also took a third group of volunteers – people who had been grossly overweight, but who had managed to slim down by near-starvation dieting. One of these, Mrs Butler, claimed she could stay slim only by limiting her intake to 600 calories a day. These people were all thin but very liable to run to fat.

The results showed that all three groups: 'fatties', 'thinnies' and 'slimmed down fatties' showed an increase in heat production immediately after a meal, but only the naturally thin group showed a substantial response. So the next question was to search for the mechanisms for this 'diet induced thermogenesis'. Could it be the result of a general increase in the rate of *all* the body's chemical processes? Was its efficiency genetically determined, or might feeding patterns in childhood set some sort of thermostat for life? Did it depend on a control system in the brain responsive to the number of fat cells in the body?

In 1979 a race was on between Dr James's group in Cambridge and a London group to find a possible mechanism. The London group were working at that time in the physiology department at Queen Elizabeth College. There, Dr Mike Stock had been hunting for a mechanism for diet-induced thermogenesis (DIT) in rats for thirteen years, and more recently had been joined by Dr Nancy Rothwell, one of his PhD students. Mike Stock's hunch was that it would be more fruitful to try to answer the question 'why do lean individuals stay lean?' rather than 'why are fat individuals fat?'

Rats were thought to provide the classic proof of theories of intake control. If parts of a rat's brain are damaged (the hypothalamus for example) it will eat uncontrollably. Normally, so it seemed, a rat would never eat an ounce more than it needed – not when offered standard laboratory chow at any rate. But Barbara Rolls in Oxford thought of tempting individual rats with delicacies, like chocolate and pork pie – lo and behold, like humans, if you give them their favourite foods they will happily over-indulge. Rats getting a varied and appetising diet like this were dubbed 'cafeteria rats'.

Mike Stock had seen the same phenomenon in his pet rat at home – so he and Nancy Rothwell decided to give their laboratory rats a similar treat. The manager of the local supermarket had no idea that the young lady filling her basket to overflowing with chocolates, crisps, ham, cakes and so on was not preparing for a huge children's party, but in fact buying food for dozens of rats.

Everything the rats consumed was weighed, and the calorific value determined by burning samples in a 'bomb calorimeter'. Many of the rats did indeed gain a lot of weight, but some individuals, like the lean people in Philip James's experiments, did not gain as much weight as expected from the amount of extra calories they had consumed. When these animals were put in calorimeters (miniature versions of the sealed rooms used at Cambridge) they consumed more oxygen than their fatter counterparts, which meant their metabolic rate had also increased in response to the extra food. So, asked Nancy Rothwell and Mike Stock, what was special about these leaner rats?

Meanwhile in Cambridge, Philip James's group was asking the question: what is special about fat people, and fat animals? Paul Trayhurn had a colony of very special mice – almost circular in shape, they are known as obob mice. They are the animal equivalents of William Campbell. Fatness does often run in families and the obob mice, like some people, are genetically programmed to become obese even on a normal diet. They are incapable of burning off surplus food.

Paul Trayhurn decided to take the temperatures of lean and obese mice to see if he could find any differences. First he took their temperatures in the animal house, which is kept quite warm. There was virtually no difference between the two types. Both groups were around 38°C. Then (and this was the beginning of a breakthrough) he took them to the cold room, where the temperature is kept at only 4°C.

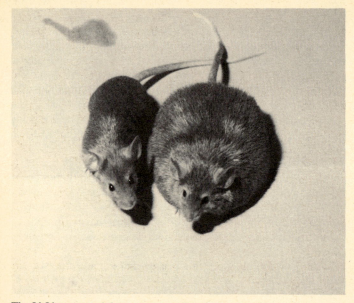

The ObOb mouse and thin companion. Genetically-obese mice are born unable to burn off surplus food. Even more interesting to the researchers, they cannot keep warm in the cold.

After two hours the lean mice had kept their temperature up at around 35°C. But the temperature of the obese mice had fallen dramatically to around 24°C. They were huddled in a corner, shivering. Paul Trayhurn was surprised. After all a fat animal is very well isulated. But these obob mice clearly could not cope with the cold, and would die soon if left in those conditions. Paul Trayhurn and Philip James were excited. Could they at last have found a method for looking at the heating processes which seem to be defective in obese individuals?

As we have seen, some of the London team's overfed 'cafeteria' rats could stay relatively slim. So how did *they* manage in the cold? Nancy Rothwell took a group of rats fed normally, and the overfed rats, and put them in the cold room. All the rats shivered at first, but after a few hours the overfed but slim group happily adapted to these wintry conditions. That also was a surprise. In adapting to an excessive intake of food, the rats had also somehow prepared themselves to cope with cold.

This is a subject fraught with apparent contradictions. Three examples: 1 If you are fat and yet do not feel the cold, this does not mean that you are actually maintaining a high body temperature in the cold. Often you feel cold precisely because your body is hotter than the surrounding air; after all you often feel cold and shivery if you have a temperature. Conversely, the colder person in some conditions feels warmer. 2 Sailors may tell you that a man overboard will survive longer in a cold sea if he is fat: that's probably because, in water, the insulating effect of the layer of fat more than makes up for his defective heating system. But fat people, like fat animals, do *not* survive better if exposed in cold air. 3 Some researchers speculate that many Americans may be overweight not because they eat too much, but because they have the central heating in their homes and offices set too high, so their bodies have no reason to burn up fat to produce heat – they do not, in other words, need to put their fat in the fire.

Some researchers had also shown that fat individuals are unable to alter metabolic rate in response either to long-term overfeeding or to a cold climate. So the London and Cambridge groups began to look through research findings on cold adaptation in animals hoping it might reveal the mechanisms involved in weight regulation.

For many years the Canadians have been studying the way both man and animals adapt to the cold. At the National Research Council near Ottawa, David Foster and Lorraine Frydman had no idea their work might become important in the study of obesity. They wanted to know just how cold-adapted animals – rats again – produce extra heat when they need it.

When you're cold, to prevent loss of heat, blood vessels just under the skin close down, and the blood flow is diverted to other parts of the body. The blood also carries with it the oxygen needed to burn fuel and produce heat. The Canadian researchers decided to compare the blood flow in animals which had been living in the warm, with those who had become adjusted to the cold. Wherever the oxygen-carrying blood went, that would be where their special furnace was.

The rats were cooled by changing the water flow around their calorimeters. As expected, their oxygen demand went up – somewhere in their bodies they were producing extra heat. Then David Foster injected radioactive microspheres into tubes already connected to the rats' hearts.

In this technique the microspheres travel down the blood vessels and jam in the tissue where the capillaries are small. The greater the number of spheres jammed in a tissue, the greater the blood flow there. David Foster, like most researchers in this field, believed the blood flow would be directed to muscle, and that this would be the site of the extra heat production.

Samples of tissue from the animals were then prepared for analysis. The final radiation count would reveal the site of the extra heat production in cold-adapted animals. Muscle tissue got a low reading. Then they checked some tissue called inter-scapular brown adipose tissue (IBAT for short, and in normal language called 'brown fat') and here, in the cold-adapted animals only, they got massively high readings. Adding the results obtained for all the brown adipose tissue in the body showed that there had been a sixty per cent rise in the amount of blood going there – almost a quarter of the total output of the heart to a very small amount of tissue. So was this where the special furnace was?

David Foster couldn't believe the results at first. With Lorraine Frydman, he checked them again and again. There was no doubt that it was brown fat. As well as greater blood flow and heat production, there also seemed to be a larger quantity of brown fat in the cold-adapted animals. So the Canadians had shown this to be the mechanism of cold adaptation. But could this special kind of fat be helping animals to stay thin as well as to keep warm?

In his years of research on diet-induced thermogenesis, Mike Stock never suspected 'in his wildest speculations' that this tissue might be involved in helping animals stay thin. But when he heard of the Canadian research he and Nancy Rothwell set out at once to check on the brown fat in their 'cafeteria' rats. Their dramatic finding was that the thinner 'cafeteria' rats had twice as much brown fat as the controls.

The Cambridge group were equally excited. If you inject noradrenaline you can artificially stimulate cells to burn their fuel stores. Paul Trayhurn injected both his fat and thin mice and measured the difference in heat production. They found that all of the differences in heat production between the two groups could be accounted for by metabolic differences in their brown fat. The cells in the brown adipose tissue of his leaner mice were burning their fuel much more fiercely.

Jean Himms-Hagen, who works in Ottawa too, is also en-thusiastic about the strange idea that brown fat may help to keep you slim. She's a biochemist who has made a special study of the tissue. Most animals have at least some brown fat, especially

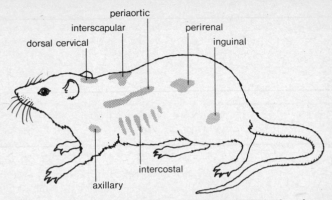

The major brown fat sites in a rat: cold-adapted and lean, food-adapted, or 'cafeteria' rats had more brown fat and burned up food more efficiently.

when young. Brown fat cells are brown, Jean Himms-Hagen told us, because they contain so many mitochondria. It is the mitochondria which actually burn the fuel and produce the heat.

She also studied a group of lean and genetically obese mice. She wanted to know if their brown fat mitochondria would differ. The Ottawa team spun homogenised brown fat tissue in a centrifuge to extract the mitochondria, then looked at them under an electron microscope. The lean mouse brown fat cells contained much bigger mitochondria.

But you can't tell just by looking at the size of the mitochondria what the secret of the burning is. That's where the biochemistry comes in. In an ordinary cell in the body, a mitochondrian is like a factory full of machines and it is designed to use energy sensibly and efficiently. But in the mitochondria in brown fat the machines are short-circuited. The energy flows through them like electricity through thousands of tiny electric fires. When the power is switched on, the heat is produced.

If all the mitochondria in your body were short-circuited like this, you would be in serious trouble. That happened to some women working in armaments factories in the First World War. In handling explosives, particularly melinite, they absorbed a chemical called dinitrophenol. This substance short-circuits mitochondria. The women became very hot indeed (one even reaching the record temperature of 109·4°F.) and they suffered acute loss of weight. In France twenty-seven such women died. Nobody at that time had any idea that there might be special cells

33

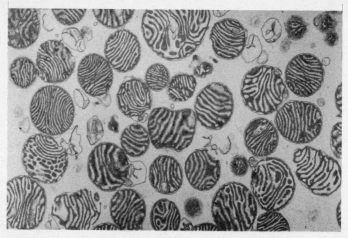

Like miniature furnaces, the mitochondria burn up fuel. Electron micrographs show that mitochondria from obese mice (below) are smaller than those in thin mice (above), and they burn up less fat.

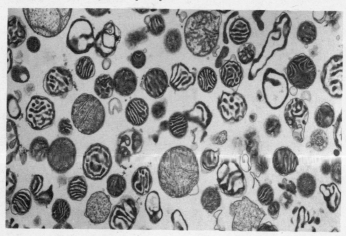

in the body containing short-circuited mitochondria which help burn up surplus food.

It was David Nicholls in Dundee who first discovered what the short-circuits in the brown fat mitochondria are made of, a protein of molecular weight 32,000 which is found *only* in brown fat. Jean Himms-Hagen found large quantities of the protein in the brown fat of both cold-adapted and lean animals. The more of this special protein there is in a cell, the more shortcircuiting goes on, and the more heat is produced. Substances called 'purine nucleotides' bind to the protein and stop the burning process. So if you measure the amount of purine nucleotide binding to the mitochondria in a piece of tissue, you can tell how well the system is functioning.

The Dunn Laboratories in Cambridge were equipped to do this kind of chemical testing, and so the rival groups decided to come together at this stage to do joint experiments. Late in 1979, Mike Stock and Nancy Rothwell took some of their 'cafeteria' rats to Cambridge. (*Horizon* had brought the two groups together over dinner one evening before filming, so perhaps we can take some credit for encouraging a kind of co-operation not all that common in science.)

They had evidence that the brown fat in their 'cafeteria-fed' rats was more active physiologically. The question was whether it would be biochemically more active too? The London rats were kept overnight in the Dunn labs, still on their diet of chocolate biscuits and pork pies. Then they were humanely killed and the brown fat dissected out. When the purine nucleotide was added, would the rats' brown fat show the same high rate of short-circuiting already shown in cold-adapted animals? The answer was yes, and a further series of experiments conducted since our film was finished have confirmed that overfed but thin rats have very effective brown fat.

So, to sum up the story so far. Fat individuals do not necess-arily eat more than thin. When thin individuals overeat they can alter their metabolic rate and burn off the surplus food. Fat individuals cannot do this and often fail to maintain body tem-perature in the cold, and so obesity and a defective heating system seem to be linked. Work in Canada on cold-adaptation in animals suggests that brown adipose tissue, or brown fat, might be the tissue where the burning up of extra food takes place. Physiological and chemical tests proved that this indeed was the site in the overfed but slim rats studied by the London group. Obese mice in Cambridge and Ottawa were found to have defective brown fat.

Both groups were very keen to find out if the same system operates in man. First Philip James took his thin, fat and slimmed-down fat patients and asked them to sit in calorimeters. He then infused noradrenaline into their bloodstreams. If brown fat or an equivalent mechanism was operating in humans, this would stimulate metabolism only in the naturally thin people as it did in Paul Trayhurn's thin mice. This is exactly what happened.

But to confirm that brown fat is the tissue involved in humans was much more difficult.

In the middle of this research, Mike Stock and Nancy Rothwell moved to St George's Hospital, Tooting. There they met Oliver Brook who had been interested for some time in calorie intake and heat production in newborn babies. Ten years before while working in Jamaica he had noticed that malnourished babies often died, not of starvation but of cold (even in that warm climate). Though brown fat was not thought significant in adults, it had been accepted for many years that very young babies use brown fat as a heating system and these babies had depleted brown fat.

Oliver Brook now studies newborns in special care units at the hospital. A newborn is so small he does not produce much heat as a byproduct of his normal body chemistry. Shivering is one emergency method the body uses to keep warm, by vibrating muscles – but a newborn cannot shiver either. Apparently he uses his brown fat as a kind of central heating system, warming the blood as it goes to the brain, heart and other vital organs in the body.

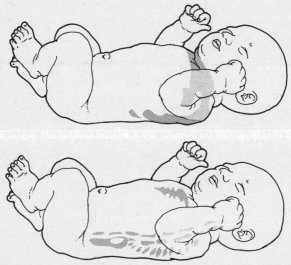

From 'The Production of Heat by Fat' by Michael J. R. Dawkins and David Hall. © 1983 Scientific American, Inc. All rights reserved.

Some of the brown fat sites in infants. The brown fat furnace keeps a newborn warm. Until the research reported by Horizon *was done, it was thought this tissue had no function in adult life.*

Oliver Brook and others have found that there is a tremendous variability both in the amount of food a baby needs to increase in size at a given rate, and in the amount of heat he produces. Also there is an increase in temperature at the brown fat sites after feeding. Long-term studies are needed next to find out if these early metabolic differences can be correlated with fatness or thinness in adult life.

One thing we already know is that it is wrong to suggest that an overfed infant will necessarily become a fat adult. If anything the reverse may be true. More recent work by Mike Stock and Nancy Rothwell reinforces this for rats: if you overfeed baby rats by the 'cafeteria' method just after weaning they turn out to be more resistant to becoming obese later in life. Their metabolic systems seem to have been put into high gear permanently. Again it seems it is not diet, not the input side, which has the most direct influence in producing obesity, but heat output and how that is controlled.

Adult humans have other heating systems, that's why it had long been assumed that they do not need to keep their infant brown adipose tissue. The quantity of the tissue declines with increasing age which reinforced the belief that it no longer plays a significant role. Nancy Rothwell decided to run a computer search through the literature for references to brown fat in adult man. She was surprised to find a very large number. And pathologists told her they found at least some brown fat in every corpse they examined. So how could one tell if this tissue had any function in adults?

Mike Stock said: 'The idea for the experiments that we undertook next came to me in a flash on a bus going over Kew Bridge. I came into the laboratory that morning and said to Nancy she was going to have to take her shirt off. I took mine off, too, and we attached temperature measuring devices all over our skin. Then we swallowed a drug which stimulates the sympathetic nervous system and so was likely to stimulate brown fat. We found very large increases in skin temperature in areas where you find brown adipose tissue. The back of the neck in particular was a site which showed large increases in temperature. This was particularly so with Nancy – but then she's much slimmer than I am!'

Mike Stock and Nancy Rothwell then decided to repeat these experiments using a thermographic camera at the Royal Marsden. The infra-red pictures revealed the sites where brown fat is usually found glowing after they took the drug. A few

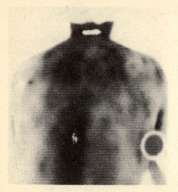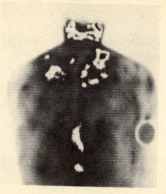

Mike Stock's back, photographed with a heat-sensitive camera, before (left) *and after* (right) *taking ephedrine to simulate the effects of eating a large meal. The brown fat sites glow brightly.*

months afterwards *Nature* published these pictures, together with a detailed report of the work with 'cafeteria' rats. Shortly before this, Philip James had published his results on the effects of noradrenalin on humans, suggesting that brown fat might be the tissue involved; and Paul Trayhurn published his work on genetically-obese mice shortly afterwards. Established authorities in the field of obesity research greeted the findings with scepticism, even hostility. The fat was in the fire.

The work with 'cafeteria' fed rats has been repeated several times, using different strains, and the results have been the same. A Dublin researcher repeated the cafeteria-feeding regime and got a sixty per cent long-term rise in metabolic rate in his rats. Jean Himms Hagen's biochemical work on mitochondria from mouse brown fat also confirmed the effect. But even so Philip James is not surprised about the scepticism. A lot more work has to be done.

He said: 'This discovery is very new indeed. In fact when *Horizon* first approached me on the subject, I said come back in a year's time. So far we've got nowhere in quantifying the significance of brown adipose tissue in humans. But the coming together now of various disparate bits of research (including ours in Cambridge, the London and Canadian work) has at the very least opened up a whole new world of experiments for us.'

Next, Philip James decided to use himself as a guineapig for particularly painful experiments at the New Addenbrooke's

Hospital in Cambridge. *Horizon* was lucky enough to be filming one of the first of these. The idea was to begin to quantify the contribution of brown fat in human thermogenesis and it was hoped to prove beyond doubt that it is an active tissue in adult humans.

First he wore a hood-calorimeter in order to monitor his oxygen uptake minute by minute. This would indicate any general increase in metabolism. A thermographic camera was surveying his back, just as in Mike Stock's experiment in London. But to get readings of temperature changes in the brown fat tissue itself, needles were inserted into Philip James's back to a depth of 2–3 inches, close to the brown fat sites, and yet other probes measured temperature in places where there is no brown fat. Then noradrenaline was infused to get the brown fat going. Sure enough, the temperature of the brown fat sites increased, while elsewhere Philip James's temperature remained

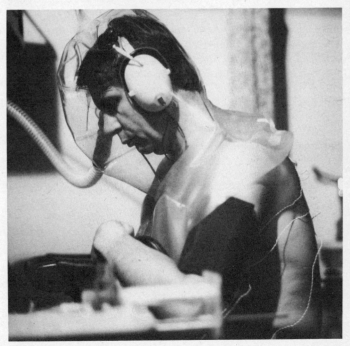

Philip James in a hood calorimeter. Temperature probes on his back registered a high reading at the brown fat sites after an injection of noradrenalin – plainly brown fat is as important in human as animal weight control.

constant or even fell. His overall metabolic rate increased. He said at the time: 'I must say, I've never had quite such a heating sensation in my life. As that noradrenaline went in one really started to burn. There was no doubt at all.'

Of course what Philip James's fat patients want to know now is how to influence the activity of the brown fat in their bodies and so allow them to eat normally and stay slim. So the hunt is now on for safe drugs which can turn on the brown fat, like the noradrenaline infused into Philip James, but in a safe and controlled way. As early as the 1930s 'reducing' drugs were marketed which caused, in the headlines of the time a 'fever that burns up fat'. Nothing was known, of course, about the special properties of brown fat, but because these substances short-circuited all the mitochondria in the body (like the dinitrophenol absorbed by those women in the First War) they disrupted a whole range of normal chemical functions and had apalling side-effects including tremor, agitation and muscle wasting. The hope is to find a way to switch on only the brown fat mitochondria, perhaps by influencing the sympathetic nervous system itself through the hypothalamus or other parts of the brain. One substance in common use appears to have this effect already: nicotine in cigarettes. Apparently that's one reason why smokers who stop put on weight. But it goes without saying that it is safer to remain overweight than to smoke so as to stay slim!

Recent research by Mike Stock and Nancy Rothwell is beginning to tease out some of the details of the system. When they have a debilitating condition called cachexia often associated with cancer, some patients literally waste away. In many cases this is not due to anorexia, as was once thought, because some sufferers continue to eat normally. In a mouse model of this cancer the London team have shown that the beta-blocker Propanolol stops this wasting effect by blocking the action of brown fat Some other drugs have a disproportionate effect on the brown adipose tissue, so Philip James is now engaged on a large scale trial to assess their effects as slimming agents.

These are only hints of things to come. It may be years before the discovery that brown fat can be an agent for weight control can be turned into safe and effective slimming treatments. Sadly the signs are that the British medical and scientific establishment will not provide the necessary funds to follow up all the new avenues of research opened up by the work done in London, Cambridge and Ottawa. Yet again a mainly British initiative may be taken up and exploited by American researchers.

Meanwhile, fatter people will have to be very patient. At least they can console themselves with the thought that most of them do not eat more than their fellows. It is just that all those smug slim people seem to be lucky enough to be born able more easily to put their excess fat in the brown fat fire.

Again, that scientific detective story does not have a neat and tidy ending. Research continues. There is much better understanding of metabolism. Some hitherto unexplained cells have taken their place in the text books. But there is no cure for obesity, and no safe slimming pill.

One of the reasons for there being few clear cut answers in medical research is that one cannot just dive with a surgeon's knife into the human body and watch cells working. Besides, they tend to stop, if you do.

The problem is greatest with brain cells. The nerve connections are so profuse the slightest damage changes the way that that part of the brain operates. Much of present knowledge about which bit of the human brain does what was reinforced by the results from the appalling number of head injuries during World War I. What the surgeons couldn't do for obvious ethical reasons, was done for them by rifle bullets and shrapnel. Soldiers hit in the back of the head went blind, others lost the ability to speak, or lost the use of certain muscles. Amidst the carnage, correlations could be made between areas of brain damage and specific disabilities. It was crude, but it confirmed and refined earlier ideas.

There is one, very common illness in which similar brain damage occurs. It is an unhappy and frustrating condition but it has provided myriads of subtle clues to the working of the body's most mysterious and delicate organ.

3 Explosions in the Mind

Robin Brightwell

The average human brain weighs just three pounds, a tiny fraction of the body's weight, yet it receives ten times its fair share of blood leaving the heart. Every minute a litre of blood flows through the complex network of arteries and veins criss-crossing the brain's surface and permeating its deepest parts. The blood carries sugar and other food constituents into every part of the brain. The nerve cells demand this nourishment for their survival: if they are deprived of blood for more than a few minutes they will die, and the individual will lose part of his or her brain function.

Sometimes in the arteries of the chest a blood clot forms. It flows easily upwards through the great arteries of the neck. But further up and deeper into the brain the vessels become increasingly narrow; the clot may stick at a junction. Nerve cells beyond receive no more blood. They starve and die. Alternatively a blood vessel may burst. Blood floods the immediate area, causes swelling and this compresses the surrounding cells, damaging them and preventing blood from reaching them through the undamaged blood vessels. So whether there is a broken or blocked vessel the effect on the individual can be instantaneous and catastrophic. We call it a stroke and it is one of the most common forms of brain damage.

The victim may be struck down just through plain bad luck, but strokes are often caused by disease to the blood system, so they are much more likely in individuals who have high blood pressure, or who are overweight, who smoke or are old. Among an average crowd of 250, as many as a dozen will have a stroke before the age of seventy. Of these twelve, six will die immediately or within a month of their stroke. Among the six survivors, two will be permanently bedridden, but the remaining four will recover to varying extents. So although strokes often cause death and permanent disability, for a third of those afflicted the outlook is not bleak. It is this more hopeful group who tell us a lot

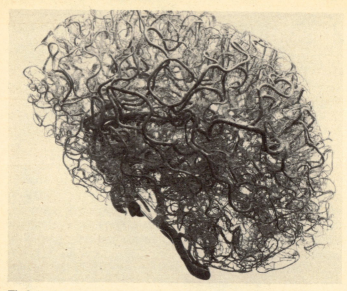

The brain is permeated by an extremely complex pattern of blood vessels. Explosions in the mind – strokes – are caused when one of them gets blocked by a blood clot, or bursts, and the surrounding nerves die.

about the brain's architecture in relation to its functions and how struggle and human determination can help restore function in the damaged areas.

If the damage is low down, in the brain centres which control breathing for example, then death will be instantaneous. Those with brain damage elsewhere, and who survive, can suffer from a whole range of effects which map the distribution of functions in the brain. They range from movement, through language, to the perception of three-dimensional space or even one's own body image.

Alistair Cameron was a banana salesman, middle-aged and comfortably off with a passion for racegoing, when a stroke paralysed his right arm and leg. His leg recovered somewhat, so he can still make it to the races, though he limps heavily. Despite his disabilities he is still determined to be jolly, and dresses in the dapper checked suit of a true 'sportsman'. Despite his paralysis, he manages to judge form through binoculars held and focused by his left hand alone. Like many victims with right-side paralysis, he has also lost much of his spoken and written language and can only place his bets by pointing out his choice to the bookie on the bookie's blackboard.

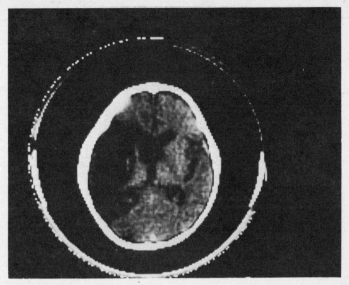

X-ray scans through the brain show up damaged areas. Here the large dark area on the left (front of head is at top of picture) means that the patient has lost much of his language and is partially paralysed.

There is a relatively new technique of brain examination called computerised axial tomography (or CAT scanning) which produces an X-ray of a slice through the brain from front to back. If Mr Cameron's brain were to be examined by CAT scanning, a dark area of dead brain would show up in the left hemisphere: the opposite side to his paralysis. The nerve fibres that used to carry and compute signals in this part of his brain no longer function. In an undamaged brain many such nerve fibres send instructions down to muscles. They start from the outside or cortex (literally the 'bark') of the brain. The fibres then pass inwards and downwards, through the centre of the brain, then further and further down towards the lower brain centres which control breathing, heart beat and digestion. These fibres gradually get closer and closer to the mid-line. Eventually they cross over from left to right and go on down into the spinal cord to link up with muscles in the right arm and leg.

It is the repertoire of signals travelling along these fibres from the *left* brain that can elicit movements on the *right* side ranging from the millimetre accuracy of a surgeon's scalpel to the simple holding of a knife. To hold a fork (in the left hand) requires in

45

addition the mirror system of control fibres crossing from the right brain to muscles on the left side. Movements of muscles in the mouth and tongue, which Mr Cameron might use, for example, to smile to order, blow out a match or eat, are controlled by a similar system split between left and right. The X-ray scan would show that he only had damage to one hemisphere so only one set of these fibres should be affected. The neat pattern of damage on the left and disability on the right does not apply throughout the body, because movements of muscles used for speech are affected by the stroke on both sides of Mr Cameron's face. This is because, in at least nine out of ten people, all language movements are controlled by the left hemisphere: hence Mr Cameron's speech problems.

The strip of brain in each hemisphere that controls all movement is parallel to and just in front of another strip which controls sensation. As a result there can be damage to one function, but not to the other; a sad situation where a patient may feel everything in a paralysed limb, yet not able to move it.

Harold Smith was one such patient. He was a sprightly seventy-five-year-old with no self-pity for his condition. Unlike Mr Cameron, his paralysis was all on the left side and although he had learnt to walk again, he could hardly move his left arm: 'I can feel everything. I can feel every touch. It doesn't matter where you touch on my arm, I can feel it, but it won't respond when I'm willing it. If something drops off the table, normally I'd have gone to pick it up but nothing happens. I just jerk forward and the arm doesn't go out to pick it.'

This frustrating effect – of feeling, but having no control of the muscles – can be even more marked, especially soon after a stroke. Dr Hamor of St Bartholomew's Hospital in London was a heart specialist who had a severe, right-hemisphere stroke one night, and was rushed unconscious to his own hospital. 'The extraordinary thing is that when I came to I felt quite normal. Its very infuriating to feel normal and part of you doesn't work. All my thought processes seemed to be normal. But it was just when I came to move the left side it wouldn't answer any of the commands. And I couldn't move about in bed freely. And there was no question of my getting up at all.'

Part of his right hemisphere had been damaged – killed off in fact. But that did not affect his thought processes. The operation of the damaged part of his brain, like so much of the brain's bulk, is unconscious in all of us. Of course, once he became accustomed to the paralysis, he began to think differently, but there was no automatic recognition within his conscious brain that part of it had been damaged beyond repair. And of course since his stroke was in the right hemisphere, his language was unaffected.

Although all right-handed people have language in their left hemisphere, there are some left-handed people who appear to have language in their right hemisphere. They do suffer from language problems after a right hemisphere stroke. But, curiously, their chances of recovery from language loss are greater. In them, language in general may be less confined to just one hemisphere.

In public Mr Cameron speaks very little; in less threatening environments his speech is better, though by no means good. It is at its best in his regular speech therapy sessions. In the following example drawn from such a session it is important to realise that he could understand the therapist perfectly well, see the pictures she was showing him, and is still a perfectly intelligent man:

> Therapist: These are some pictures with 'f' sounds in. Can you tell me what this picture is?
> Mr Cameron: Er . . . fi-fish.
> Therapist: A fish, yes. Could you give me a sentence with that word in it?
> Mr Cameron: Fish – er . . .
> Therapist: What would you say?
> Mr Cameron: Um . . .
> Therapist: Where is it, where is . . .
> Mr Cameron: Oh . . . sea
> Therapist: Sea, so – the
> Mr Cameron: Seaside . . .
> Therapist: So – the – fish – is
> Mr Cameron: is on
> Therapist: in
> Mr Cameron: in – the water
> Therapist: Good – the fish is in the water.

Mr Cameron's problem is not in operating or controlling his muscles, as we know from his competence at eating, smiling, laughing and so on. He is using many of the same muscles then as he does for speech. So he really does have a disorder of language, not just of speech. For example, he can often find the appropriate noun, but cannot speak in sentences. He cannot, by himself, use the 'functional' words of grammar: verbs, prepositions, articles, endings. In the example above he has to be given a lot of prompting to use 'the', 'is', 'on'. For such patients the most difficult phrase to repeat is, 'No "ifs", "ands" or "buts"': to them it means nothing. They cannot discover the words from the sounds, even though they hear them. Similarly, they cannot construct the sounds as normal individuals can: they have lost the apparatus for creating conventional sentences. This disability of Mr Cameron is related to the site of his stroke damage. Similar patients have been examined by a novel technique developed by Drs Ingvar and Lassen in Copenhagen.

A harmless radioactive tracer is injected into an artery in the neck, which supplies the left hemisphere. Blood flow distributes the isotope throughout the brain, and it is washed through fastest where the brain is working hardest. If an area is damaged, little or no blood flows through and it shows up black. Patients with language disabilities like Mr Cameron's show black areas of damage in a particular part of the left hemisphere towards the front. This is called Broca's area after Paul Broca, the French doctor who discovered it in 1861. It is just in front of those parts of the cortex which control movements of the right limbs, which explains why right-side paralysis and this language defect are associated in Mr Cameron and many others. Their language is often described as 'telegrammatic', and indeed it does have some of the curt character of a telegram; but their frustration is well beyond any felt by the normal person trying to compress their message into the space of a few brief words. Very often one feels that the patient wishes to communicate something, knows what it is, but cannot say it. The puzzle remains: are the words in there and he is trying to get them out or are they just 'not there'. We can never be sure, as the victim cannot tell us – but evidence suggests that the desire to communicate is there, the words are not.

Another group of stroke victims have no trouble speaking in full sentences, and to a casual listener sound impressively articulate. Yet on analysis, their speech and their writing convey little meaning: it's like a 'word salad'. One patient was asked to describe a picture showing two boys stealing biscuits behind a woman's back and said: 'Mother is away here working her work to get her better, but when she's looking the two boys looking in the other part. She's working another time.'

When this second group of patients are examined with the Copenhagen machine, damage usually shows up again on the left side, in support of Broca's original findings, but the affected part is further back than Broca's area. It is named Wernicke's area,

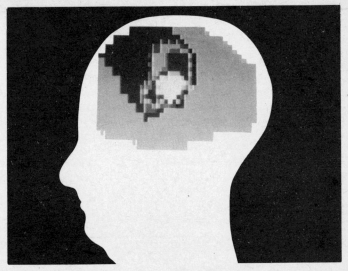

By measuring blood flow through the brain, damaged areas can be mapped. When results from several patients with Broca's Aphasia were pooled, all had damage in the white area in the middle, which shows an association between the disability and the area damaged.

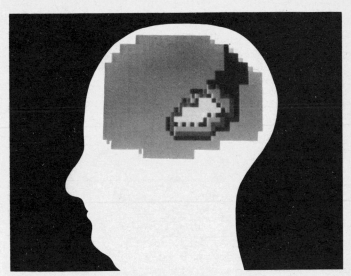

Other patients show common damage in a different area because their language disorder, called Wernicke's Aphasia, is also different.

49

after its German discoverer. It is adjacent to the terminus for nerve fibres coming from the ears and indeed there does seem to be some connection between the patients' strange language and their inability to check and analyse their own or others' speech. Normal speech involves a continual quality control check. We know that takes place because of the unnerving experience of having one's own voice played back through head phones with a second or so's delay. They lack the ability to check accurately what they are saying, and as a result their own language goes all over the place. Similarly they have trouble understanding normal speech. Their analysis of sound input has been destroyed by the stroke and this also destroys their ability to choose the appropriate words. Yet this does little to explain their language disorder in detail. Likewise the explanation for the activity of Broca's area is no more detailed: it encodes language for speech or writing. The grammatical errors and deficits of someone with brain damage in Broca's area are a mystery. For example, when presented with the spoken sentence 'The lion was killed by the tiger', those with damage in Broca's area typically cannot answer the question: 'Which animal died?'! This is, once again, because they cannot understand the grammar. To them the sentence becomes: 'Buzz lion buzz killed buzz buzz tiger'. Clearly, understanding only the nouns does not make clear which animal died. We have no idea how the brain actually does analyse such questions in normal people.

All we know is the likely connections between various areas. For example, if someone hears a spoken word, and is asked to repeat it, the sound goes in through the ear, reaches the adjacent section of the brain, the auditory cortex, where the sounds are analysed and sent on to Wernicke's area. From there the nerve signals travel forward to Broca's area, where as we know some form of grammatical analysis takes place, then back a little to the motor cortex where movements are designed and from where instructions are sent down to the spinal cord and so to the muscles of the lips and tongue for speech.

Our sketchy knowledge of language and its relationship to the brain is reflected in the treatment of language disorders. Speech therapy undoubtedly helps recovery, often months or even years after a stroke or other brain damage, but this may merely be because the patient is forced to practise speaking and is given encouragement. It is not because of any specific pattern to the therapy based on a theory. For the patient all that matters of course is that recovery does take place, but therapists would

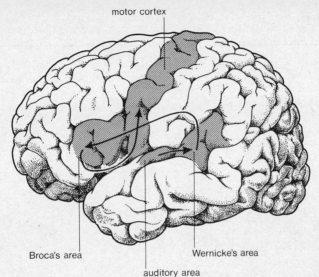

motor cortex

Broca's area   Wernicke's area

auditory area

Sounds travel, as nerve impulses, to the auditory cortex for initial deciphering. They pass to Wernicke's area, in the left hemisphere, then to Broca's area, for conversion into a form suitable for speech, then to the part which controls speech movements.

dearly love to have a more effective method with a theory to back it up and so to extend it. That may not occur until we understand the relationship between language and the brain in more detail than we do now.

If the left hemisphere controls language, except in a small proportion of left-handers, then what does the right hemisphere do? Many functions exist on both sides: movement, all the senses, memory, planning ahead, and so on. The right hemisphere seems to be more musical in adults and often someone with a severe language disability and only able to speak the occasional word, will still be able to sing a song, including all the words, for verse after verse. The intact musical ability is his right hemisphere somehow provides a rhythmic framework and enables the singer to form words despite damage in the normal language areas. Also the right hemisphere deals with spatial skills, as another stroke victim, Peter Leuw, so clearly demonstrates.

He was a British Airways Executive, but several years ago he was forced to retire. His stroke was in the right hemisphere, and occurred while he was on business in Australia. He was rushed back to London, and in Charing Cross Hospital the strange pattern of his disabilities began to unfold.

It affected even something as basic as putting on his clothes. When picking up garments he found it impossible to tell front from back, and if left to himself would often struggle to put them on the wrong way round. Clothes often have a maker's label attached inside the collar. Finding this a help, he asked his wife to mark all his clothes similarly. This device didn't always work, so they tried the trick of leaving his clothes always face down, so that he would know immediately which side was the back.

The extraordinary thing was that nevertheless a struggle would take place in Peter's brain as to which side was front and which back. Despite what his brain was telling him, the necessities of everyday life insisted that he believe instead what his wife told him. The effort to do so sometimes made him giddy. As Peter said: 'Even despite the sweater being marked, the struggle went on in my mind to put it on back to front. My mind or brain was saying "Put it on back to front," but something else in me was saying, "Now don't be silly, you can't do it that way. You won't half look silly walking down the street with a tie dangling down your back." You know this sort of thing, and you just had to push on and do it that way.'

The right parietal lobe of the brain, which is about halfway back, normally enables us to build an internal 'model' or framework of our bodies, and the three-dimensional spaces – the environment – into which they fit. This had been destroyed in Peter Leuw, and he had to use a series of rules, such as the label on the back of cardigans, shirts and so on, to enable him to dress correctly. There were other unpleasant surprises to come: 'Carrol asked me to make out a cheque and she came back and said "You've made it out upside down." I was a little terse about this, because it's a pretty difficult thing to make a cheque out upside down. So I said, "Well what's wrong?" And she said, "It's just simply upside down." And she went to one of the consultants who was very excited about the whole thing and said, "Well, he's got this left side inattention." I don't know what medical term they used at the time, and then a very charming psychologist came along and did some tests on me and they asked me to do various things and only then it became apparent to me in the hospital that I'd got this "trouble"'.

One particularly noticeable symptom was, that as far as Peter

Leuw's brain was concerned, the left side of objects, and the left side of his own body did not exist. His brain ignored them.

He could no longer map-read: 'I was asked in the hospital, after being an RAF navigator and being very involved in flying as a career, to draw a map of Britain. I went gaily about it: and then when I looked at it, or they, the medicos did, they said "Look you've left out the whole of the left side of Britain. There is no Wales." And what really hurt me, I had even left out the Isles of Scilly, with which I was very involved, and still am with the helicopter service out there. I had overlooked Cornwall naturally. No Isles of Scilly, therefore no helicopters, which really hurt me. Now I think I can do a little bit better, I can even map-read a little now.'

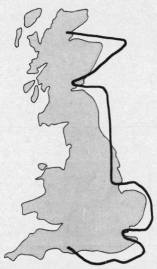

After his right-hemisphere stroke, Peter Leuw was asked to draw the map of England. The heavy line shows what he drew: the whole left side of the country was left out. But he remembered the east coast fairly accurately.

Patients more disabled than Peter Leuw, with paralysis as well, often have terrible difficulties deciding how to put clothes on. A young mother with such disabilities, Penney Culley, spent an agonising five minutes trying to put a pair of tights on her baby. She continually put the baby's left leg into the wrong leg of the tights and could not comprehend the spatial relationship between the baby and his clothes.

Now Peter Leuw and his wife live in a cottage in Somerset. His movements are normal, as are his speech and appearance. But ask him to copy a pattern of eight matches arranged in a star shape and the result is both sad and fascinating for the observer, and terribly frustrating for him. He can copy simpler shapes, like a square of four matches, with no difficulty.

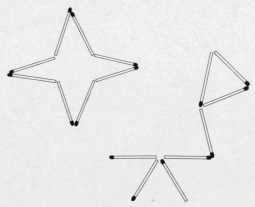

When asked to arrange 8 matches in a star shape (as left), the best Peter Leuw could manage, despite many frustrating attempts, was the shape on the right.

The patterns of stroke damage do not enable us to distinguish all major functions of each hemisphere, only those which reflect the distribution of blood vessels. The parts of the brain which are killed are those fed by the blood vessels most likely to become blocked, or most likely to haemorrhage.

Apart from those few cases where surgery can provide a by-pass for the blood supply, there is no medical way to restore the damaged brain to normal. Yet natural recovery does take place, though it is slow and often incomplete. That process is still a puzzle; and, although medicine attempts to restore stroke victims to as normal a life as possible, it is only sometimes successful.

That success can be fairly quick. If there was a blockage the brain often swells and this is the usual cause of death soon afterwards in strokes caused by blocked vessels. If the swelling can be reduced by drugs the patient may survive, but be left with a central core of dead nerve cells, and a surrounding 'shadow' of inactive, but still living cells. These may recover normally or under the influence of certain drugs which enhance the brain's natural ability to re-supply the tissue with blood. Such reawakening brain cells are the cause of recovery in the first few weeks.

The truly dead cells can never be revived. That may not always matter because many parts of the brain can be removed or killed with relatively little loss of function.

However, strokes are one of the major causes of disability in middle and old age, and have been for many years. It is therefore, at first sight, surprising that the long term treatment of stroke patients is so unsatisfactory in many hospitals. For example, until recently even enlightened hospitals assigned stroke victims to the care of specialists in 'rheumatology' – doctors concerned with the treatment of rheumatism and arthritis. Consequently no valid theory has yet been developed to point to an overall strategy for the treatments of those paralysed by strokes, and patients have often been neglected. A few centres are gradually developing more sophisticated techniques based on the knowledge we now have about brain damage and its particular characteristics, rather than the damage to body joints which characterises rheumatism and arthritis.

For example, recovery from strokes continues for months, and occasionally for years. The language of Mr Cameron, the racegoer, is still slowly improving. Others suddenly gain the partial use of their arm or leg up to two years after the stroke. If dead cells are not being revived other mechanisms must enable the immensely complex patterns of nerves to operate. Suddenly they can process signals in a new way, and pass them on to the identical muscles. If only we knew how to maximise this ability, many sad lives would be transformed. Some hospitals and rehabilitation centres spend a lot of effort on physiotherapy, speech therapy and the like to do just this and they do often prevent the worst effects of stroke, such as the contortions of spastic limbs. They certainly also keep the patients' spirits up, but the therapists do not know why their treatments work, and they would be the first to admit that frequently they do not work.

It would help if we knew what happens during long-term recovery. Research in other fields suggests a range of explanations for it. Sarah Hearn used to be a home-brewing enthusiast, but a few years ago a demijohn she was washing shattered, and the glass cut her wrist, severing a major nerve. The flesh wound healed rapidly but she had lost all sensation in her fingertips. Although the muscles were unaffected, her hand would not do up buttons, open tins, or do needlework and she could not write very well. Fortunately the hospital were able, by minor surgery, to provide a tunnel for the nerve to grow through. Over the months, it reached her thumb and fingers and gradually Mrs Hearn felt more and more tingling in her fingers, as the nerve fibres were once again able to pass signals from skin to brain. This was not, of course, the revival of a dead brain cell. But in the brain, cells do 'branch' or 'sprout' in a similar way and this may gradually restore function after stroke. The new growth may be long enough to bridge and by-pass areas of damage. Mrs Hearn needed months of extensive retraining, practising detailed finger movements, before function was restored. So retraining, by speech therapy or certain repetitive movements of limbs in physiotherapy, may do the same for stroke victims. Recent clinical trials suggest that any such effect is often completely swamped by the family doing too much, indeed often doing everything for their handicapped relative, so he or she gets no practice of speech or movement at home.

There is an alternative recovery mechanism, best illustrated by Vicky Hughes, who was only six when she had her stroke. She couldn't speak and X-rays confirmed that the stroke was in her left hemisphere. Damage there had destroyed her language skills. As the months passed, very surprisingly her language gradually returned. After eighteen months of recovery, she could sing and dance and showed little handicap on her affected right side. Her speech was not yet normal, but it was fluent. When a series of recordings were made of the electrical activity on the skin of her head, reflecting the brain's activity beneath, the left hemisphere still showed reduced activity, as it had for the previous eighteen months, but her right hemisphere had become much more active. The conclusion, supported by other cases like Vicky's, is that the right hemisphere does have the capacity to carry out all language functions, but is normally suppressed by the more dominant language abilities of the left side of the brain. It takes some months for the right side to express itself, but in some young children it certainly can. We do not know if Vicky and other such children are typical, but the ability to transfer language spontaneously definitely declines with age.

Some research scientists, such as Dr Tony Buffery at the Institute of Psychiatry in London, believe it may be possible to train adult stroke victims to speak, read and write with their right hemispheres. If the right side is trained by receiving speech through tape recordings fed to the left ear, and words projected onto the left visual field, it may come into its own. The work is at an early stage, so it is too soon to say whether this technique holds any hope for Alistair Cameron and the thousands of others who lose their language from strokes every year.

Doctors in the field, like Dr Dennis Smith from Northwick Park Hospital, admit that, help though they may, stroke recovery is not in their hands alone. He believes that the most important factor is whether a patient is motivated towards making a recovery. If he or she is intelligent and had a lot of drive before-hand, then all efforts are quite likely to be put into making a good recovery. Even though someone's disability may be high, func-tional recovery may be much better than in someone who is poorly motivated towards getting better.

One of the many people who illustrate this is Harold Smith. He is a sprightly old man who obviously fell into the category that his namesake Dr Smith identified as those most likely to make the best possible recovery. His leg has recovered well enough so that he can now hobble about, but his left arm is still useless. Fortunately language is unaffected and he certainly does not feel sorry for himself: 'At seventy-five you don't expect to start get-ting up and learning how to walk, but I managed, without a stick, so I don't worry any more. I just say to myself probably in time this arm will come right. Perhaps it won't. I shan't worry. If it does I shall be very thankful.'

The success in stroke therapy has been remarkable. Better understanding of the damage in individual cases has been combined with the recognition of the need for speed. The therapist can now begin specific brain exercises, which usually means body exercises, at a very early stage. The other important factor is the personality of the individual. Strong characters do well, weak ones less well.

But what do adjectives describing personality mean? Where does personality come from? Although there has been some argument, it is now generally agreed that the brain is purely a chemical machine. Whatever it is that makes humans individual personalities, it is some combination of brain chemicals. New ones are being discovered all the time. The latest, which has been called tribulin, seems to be connected with fear and panic. But the discovery of the endorphins, which appear to control pain and to blot out other unpleasant experiences, was one of the most unusual and exciting stories in the history of biochemistry – especially for the young scientists involved.

4 The Keys of Paradise

Dick Gilling

The path of scientific discovery is not as straight as a Roman road. It is more like a footpath through hilly, wooded country: sometimes in dark, overgrown places, prickly with bramble bushes; sometimes in dappled shade, offering glimpses into other sunlit clearings; very occasionally emerging at the top of a hill to reveal the pattern of the countryside. Sometimes, when an idea's time has come, it turns out that several people have been following their different, tortuous paths which have led to the same scenic outlook. That is what happened in this story.

The objective towards which the scientists thought they were heading was the discovery of the biochemical basis of drug addiction. Since narcotic drugs are simply chemicals of one sort or another, it seems reasonable to suppose that addiction to them is the result of some interference with the chemistry of the body. The scientists were looking for the details of this process, with the idea that it should be possible to interrupt whatever stage it was that caused addiction.

There was an urgent necessity for such a medical programme in the late Sixties, particularly in the United States. One of the unexpected results of the conflict in Vietnam and the ground-swell of opposition to it was a huge increase in the habit of taking narcotic drugs, particularly the opiates. Opium itself, of course, is an ancient drug. Many people in nineteenth-century Britain were addicted to it, it was almost as freely available as tobacco, and not regarded much differently. The poet Thomas de Quincey, a self-confessed 'opium eater', wrote the lines from which the title of this chapter is taken:

'Thou hast the Keys of Paradise, O just, subtle, and mighty Opium!'

More recently, Graham Greene has written of smoking opium during his frequent travels in Indo-China and of its pleasures. But the self-destructive quality of the habit, too, has always been known. In a desperate attempt to prevent the import of opium by

British traders, the Chinese fought a war in the nineteenth century, and lost. The soldiers in Vietnam found themselves lonely, bored and frightened, and loose in a country where the opium poppy was a staple crop and opiate drugs were available in vast quantities; so they availed themselves. When they went home they took the habit with them and the traffic followed. The increase in drug addiction alarmed even the U.S. authorities, who had been struggling with the trade in illegal narcotics for years.

It was impossible simply to prohibit the trade. The experiment of prohibition of alcohol had been a major disaster, and anyway the opiate drugs like morphine and heroin were far too important for the alleviation of pain. There are still no convincing substitutes for them. If, however, the problem of addiction could be solved at its biochemical roots, at least there would be the hope of a reliable treatment. The President, Richard Nixon, announced the allotment of very large funds to solve the problem.

The opiates are not merely painkillers. They also depress respiration and lower blood pressure, as well as inducing constipation and impotence; rather fortunately, in the circumstances, they also induce a feeling of well-being – euphoria. Quite evidently, their actions are widespread and complex. It seemed best to look for a site of activity in the central nervous system – specifically in the brain.

President Nixon's dollar windfall settled in many places. One of them was the Addiction Research Foundation at Palo Alto, south of San Francisco, where a leading pharmacologist, Avram Goldstein, is the Director. Goldstein's first strategy was to find a receptor for the morphine molecule on the brain cell. No one has yet seen a receptor or is quite sure what they ought to look like; but in current biochemical thinking, a receptor is a molecule, located on the membrane surrounding a cell, which is like a keyhole in which other chemical molecules – in this case morphine – fit. Once the specific key molecule has found the keyhole (or receptor) molecule, the cell is by some means activated to perform some function, here depressing pain signals.

Goldstein knew that morphine molecules come in two kinds, which relate as a left hand and a right hand relate: mirror images of each other. The property is not unique to morphine. The right-handed molecule is totally inert; it is the left-handed molecule that is active. 'It was on that basis,' says Goldstein, 'that we set out to discover where in the brain was the binding site of these molecules that had the right shape: sites that would not bind the wrong shape. And that became the basis eventually for the opiate receptor binding assays that are now used widely all over the world.'

Goldstein described his idea, and suggested how the research might be conducted, in 1971. But by a rather unkind quirk of fate, his laboratory was not the one to find the receptor.

The experiment was not easy. If a brain cell were to be enlarged to the size of a city, the receptor molecule would be about the size of a keyhole on a door in a house in the city. It was almost certain to be found, if it existed at all, in the area of the nerve cell where messages from one cell are transmitted to another, the synapse. At that point, a fibre from one cell almost but not quite touches a fibre from another. Each cell may have thousands of synapses. At these near-junctions, signals are passed in the form of chemicals, known as neuro-transmitters, and here, or so there was every reason to think, would also be found the morphine receptors. So tiny are the synapses that they can only be clearly seen under the electron microscope. No form of micro-surgery could isolate them, but there is a method that can do this. Brain cells are homogenised into a thin soup with a

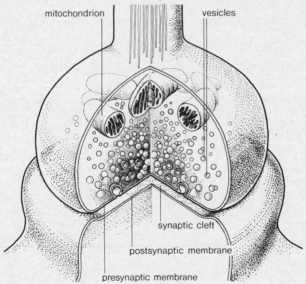

From 'The Neuron' by Charles F. Stevens. © 1983 Scientific American, Inc. All rights reserved.

The Synapse: The vesicles of the upper cell contain neuro-transmitters which travel through the presynaptic membrane and across the synaptic cleft to influence the postsynaptic membrane.

61

particular chemical, and spun in a centrifuge, separating the constituents by weight so that the part of the soup containing the synapses can be drawn off. However carefully the job is done, it is a messy business, and the purified synapse material may be easily contaminated with unwanted bits of cell. Then, one has to persuade morphine molecules to attach themselves firmly into the receptor molecules (always assuming there are any) and, the neatest trick of all, prove that the active, left-handed molecules are thus firmly bound.

The accepted method for establishing this proof is itself ticklish, though simple enough in principle. A radioactive atom is attached to each morphine molecule, and the morphine mixed with the synapse material; the mixture is 'washed' to remove any unbound morphine, and put into a machine which measures radioactivity; appropriate signals of radioactivity will reveal morphine bound to the synapses, and hence the presence of morphine receptors. But, alas, more than a waving of hands and a quick 'hey presto!' were needed for this particular piece of magic.

Several laboratories were anxious to be first in the race to find the morphine receptor. After a number of fruitless attempts, Goldstein even published a paper suggesting that the receptor site did not exist, which he would later regret. A Swedish scientist at the University of Uppsala, Lars Terenius, who had been working on steroid receptors was particularly well equipped; so were Eric Simon, in New York, and Solomon Snyder, at Johns Hopkins in Baltimore. One point all three picked up from Goldstein's paper: his laboratory was using a rather weakly radioactive morphine-like molecule. One way of getting results would be to make the radioactive molecule 'hotter'.

Nice guys, it has been said, finish last. As it happened, the race to find the morphine receptor was pretty well the scientific equivalent of a photo-finish. The winner by a short head was in Snyder's laboratory in Baltimore; at the time she was a graduate student who was putting a lot of work into repeated experiments. Her name is Candace Pert.

'It was the last experiment I did one Friday,' she said. 'I picked my little boy up from nursery school because it got late, and came back to the laboratory with him. He helped me cap the vials and put them into the counter.'

Candace Pert went home for a family weekend, and left the automated radioactivity counter to its own devices over the two days till Monday. She wasn't expecting much.

'Monday morning I came in and got the counts and sat down at my desk to look them over. As I was copying the numbers down I couldn't believe that it was working out so beautifully, and my friend, Ann Young, sitting at the next desk, said, "What's the matter?" and I said, "Do you know where the nearest bar is?" She said, "Is it that bad, is it that awful? Do you need to get drunk?" I said, "No, I want to buy a bottle of champagne. I can't believe that it worked!" and I showed it to her, and she was the first one to see the results, and we were very excited.'

Pert had been using a very 'hot' radioactivity, and very thorough washing techniques learned from an endocrinologist in a neighbouring laboratory. She had also used not morphine or a morphine analogue, but a morphine antagonist, naloxone, which was to play a large part in the story as a whole. Naloxone attaches itself to the morphine receptor molecule even more strongly than morphine itself; so strongly, indeed, that it actually displaces the morphine molecule. Developed to bring round victims of opiate overdose (which it can do in as little as thirty seconds) it was an invaluable tool, not only in Candace Pert's research but in research yet to come.

The two other competitors announced their results only days later. Since three respected laboratories, Snyder's, Simon's and Terenius's, all had come to essentially the same conclusion, it was now accepted that there was indeed a receptor molecule, a keyhole, for morphine, and that it was to be found on the brain cell.

The scene now shifts to Britain – or, more specifically to Scotland. In Aberdeen, Hans Kosterlitz, a pharmacologist, was nearing retirement when the Nixon dollars enabled him to start a Unit for Research on Addictive Drugs as part of the University. Kosterlitz and another pharmacologist, Harry Collier of Miles Laboratories in Stoke Poges, had discussed the possibility of a morphine receptor together. A striking idea had come to both of them, before the receptor had been even found; it was an idea so simple, but so profound, that many others in the field were to claim it, perhaps because it seems in retrospect quite obvious. Why, they thought, would there be a receptor in the brain for poppy-juice? Surely it must be that the brain had its own poppy-juice: a key which would fit the lock of the receptor molecule. Such coincidence between plant and animal compounds was not unknown: the tobacco leaf's nicotine mimics the neurotransmitter acetylcholine, and ephedrine, from a desert shrub, mimics noradrenaline. The next phase of the hunt was up.

Like jokes, new scientific ideas often turn up through the connection of several components, some of which may be likely and
others totally unlikely. While Snyder, Terenius and the others
were mincing their rat brains and measuring radioactivity to find
out facts at a molecular level, another group of young researchers in California were looking at behaviour. This group,
Huda Akil, John Liebeskind and David Mayer, was specifically
engaged at the time in research on pain; of course, they would be
interested in morphine; of course they had followed the argu-
ments about the morphine receptor (Pert and Snyder's discovery
had not yet been published) and had picked up the idea that
there might be some kind of opiate substance already in the
brain. Ideas were already spreading quickly at international conferences.

Huda Akil had been working with rats which had electrodes
implanted in their brains in a location where electrical stimulation can 'switch off' or at least reduce sensitivity to pain. This is
now becoming a well-known surgical procedure in humans for
use in cases where pain-killing drugs no longer work; it is an
extremely delicate operation, and research like Huda Akil's has
helped to make it acceptably safe and effective. However, pain
research on rats does mean that at some time, the rat has to be
hurt to find out whether he feels any pain. Akil used a well-
established test to find out how well the brain electrodes worked.
It simply consisted of applying heat from a small light-bulb to the
rat's tail, and timing the interval before he moved it away from
the heat: the so-called tail-flick test. One curious effect the team
(and others) had noticed about this electrical analgesia was that it
gradually reduced in efficiency: the animals became habituated
to the stimulation just as they did to pain-killing drugs like
morphine. Two very different methods of pain relief had this
common feature. Why? The team discussed various ideas.
Maybe both systems used the same chemical in the brain to kill
the pain somehow; perhaps by switching off selected nerve
signals at the synapse, which used chemical transmitters anyway?
Perhaps.

One night Huda Akil decided to test out one of the ideas they
had discussed. This was to see whether naloxone, which would
nullify the effects of morphine, would also nullify the effects of
the electrodes. It didn't seem very likely, but why not try it on
just one rat?

'So I stayed on one evening late and thought I would try this
one animal, and find out; and I did it, and it worked. I thought, 'I

don't believe it,' and so I did another animal, then another animal, and I ended up doing the whole study that evening. I was very thrilled and at the same time I kept thinking, well, maybe there is another explanation . . .'

The rest of the team heard about it the next day; Huda Akil had been too tired to ring them up the previous night. Over the next few days they ran the tests again in different ways, using controls, and came up with the same results. So they wrote a paper and sent it off for publication.

Another member of the group, David Mayer, looked round for some way in which a similar effect could be shown on people. Ethical problems would prevent his using patients with implanted electrodes; and no one could be asked to volunteer to have electrodes implanted. After casting about, he settled on acupuncture. It was becoming clear that acupuncture did give relief from pain in a considerable number of patients; since it is reve·sible and free from side effects, though most doctors are probably sceptical of it, it still seemed Mayer's best bet. He designed an experiment in which pain would be induced by touching a volunteer's tooth with an electric probe; an acupuncturist would then abolish the pain – or try to – and Mayer would administer naloxone to see if the pain came back.

Of course, the experiment worked. Mayer was delighted, but a little embarrassed that he would be obliged to offer as evidence a procedure – acupuncture – which was equated in many quarters with black magic. But the results did seem to offer the required evidence, however indirect, that a mechanical procedure which reduced pain was operating through a chemical medium, since its effects could be reversed chemically. Whether anyone could be persuaded to take them seriously was another matter.

Meanwhile, in Aberdeen, Hans Kosterlitz was after the real thing: the brain's own morphine, which he now felt sure existed. As it turned out, finding it was a task that made cleansing the Augean stables look like dusting a bedroom.

The first necessity was to get hold of enough material to examine; in short, brains. The team settled on pig brain, which could be got hold of fairly easily – and reasonably cheaply. Since there was no clear idea of what sort of chemical they might be looking for, there was not much option except to try to purify as many substances as possible and test them to see whether they behaved in any way like morphine. John Hughes was the man largely responsible for carrying out this part of the research programme; he had to find a test which was sensitive and reliable enough to tell him unequivocally whether any of the extracts was indeed morphine-like.

The usual test at the time for morphine-like compounds involved using part of a guinea-pig intestine. Morphine is known to have effects on gut: part of its use in medicine is to prevent unwanted bowel contractions. By stimulating the isolated piece of guinea-pig gut electrically, it could be made to contract; morphine (*or* a morphine-like compound) would stop the contractions; naloxone would reverse that effect. Up to that time the guinea-pig test had been widely used and pretty successful, but Hughes decided to introduce a different piece of tissue into the test. A student of his, Graham Henderson, had been using mouse vas deferens (a tiny duct that carries the spermatozoa from the testes to the sperm sac) in pharmacological tests; by substituting this for the guinea-pig gut, Hughes believed he would get a more sensitive test. That turned out to be right.

Hughes and his colleagues spent six months purifying extracts from pig brain and testing them, quite without success. Then their luck turned, as John Hughes said: 'Usually when we collected fractions and they proved negative, the stuff was put away in the deep freeze. It so happens that about six months after we started the project we started to clear out the deep freeze, and the technician asked me if she should throw them away. I thought, well, perhaps we'd better check them again. And a couple of bottles that had proved negative before turned out this time to be positive. One of the jokes in the laboratory at the time was "Have you checked that no one's been storing morphine next to your flasks in the fridge?" But the reason why the extracts were positive was very simple. When you store substances in the fridge, some things go off faster than others, and fortunately the active substance was fairly stable under those conditions.'

The mixture of compounds that Hughes had extracted, had more or less purified itself in the fridge. Without this convenient and unlooked-for accident, Hughes and Kosterlitz might still be looking. As it was, they named the substance 'enkephalin', meaning 'in the head'. And they felt confident enough to announce their findings at a conference in America.

Huda Akil remembers the occasion vividly: 'The level of excitement and electricity was almost palpable; People were talking beforehand about the fact that they thought that John Hughes and Hans Kosterlitz were going to announce that they had a substance which was natural to the brain and would affect the opiate receptor – somehow the news had been leaked. Then

John Hughes presented his material, and he was very measured about it, very scientific and calm and gave his data, and it was very nice and convincing. And people were extremely excited, I thought, and were really trying to find out more, and he didn't know any more.'

What Hughes did not know, in common with everyone else, was what enkephalin actually was. It had a name, but its chemical composition was still unknown. Even its existence was doubted, specifically by the publisher of the journal to which Hughes sent his report: 'The first paper went back and forth between the editor and myself, I think two or three times. I was greeted by rank disbelief on his part.'

As it happens, Lars Terenius had suggested at the conference that enkephalin might be a peptide – a long chain-molecule made up from a number of amino-acids, and quite a different sort of structure from morphine. Terenius turned out to be correct, but what Hughes now needed was to establish which amino acids were involved, and which order they were assembled in: the order is crucial for the molecule's chemical activity. That work took almost another year, during which Kosterlitz and Hughes were uncomfortably aware that several other laboratories, including Terenius's and Snyder's, were also trying to get to the finishing post first.

The Aberdeen group now needed much larger quantities of the brain material, and help on an almost industrial scale with its purification. The amount of enkephalin in one brain was minute: almost literally a drop in an ocean. And the analysis would need much more than the laboratory could supply on its own. They enlisted the help of one pharmaceutical company, but for reasons they choose not to discuss, parted after a short time. Then Kosterlitz visited Reckitt and Colman in Hull, and they agreed to help. Barry Morgan, of Reckitt's, got hold of a huge supply of pig brains from a local abattoir, and did the initial purification in Hull. He was using industrial equipment, and at one stage alarm bells rang, metaphorically, when he thought that the brain extract carried traces of one of Reckitt's better-known household products, Brasso. The huge vat the brains were being processed in was normally used for that metal polish; but it was a false alarm. After months of effort, there was enough enkephalin available for the Aberdeen team, with Barry Morgan's help, to start on a biochemical analysis in earnest.

Linda Fothergill, in Aberdeen, was able before very long to identify the first four amino acids in order; but after the fourth, she ran into trouble, and so did everyone else. It was clear that others were involved – maybe half a dozen others – and Fothergill and Morgan's methods did not seem to be capable of sorting the muddle out.

One of the few people able to help was Howard Morris, then at the MRC Pharmacology unit in Cambridge. Hughes gave a seminar there in the spring of 1975, in the course of which he mentioned the problem he had. Morris offered to help with his own technique of mass spectroscopy; but Hughes gave him at the time, says Morris, 'a rather abrupt answer that the chemists in Aberdeen had advised him that this was only useful for confirming structures, not establishing them and so I didn't pursue the matter at that stage.'

Barry Morgan, meanwhile, had been searching through the literature, and had decided that the very man to help was – Howard Morris. He arranged to attend a meeting in London where Morris would be speaking, and afterwards approached Morris, who once again offered to help. A week or so later, a few precious microgrammes of the material came down from Aberdeen, and Morris started on his part of the work.

The evidence so far suggested that enkephalin was a peptide containing eight or ten amino acids. Morris, with his special technique rather quickly found a pentapeptide – one with five amino acids. The sequence was: Tyrosine, Glycine, Glycine, Phenylalanine, Methionine. He rang Barry Morgan, who at once began to synthesise the peptide. This was a necessary step; if the synthetic material behaved like the natural extract, the team could be pretty sure they were on the right track. Next day, Morris rang Morgan again in a state of some excitement: he had found another pentapeptide in the material, with the first four places in the sequence the same, but the last place occupied by Leucine. The sample had contained not one long peptide, but two shorter ones. And the material Morgan synthesised had exactly the effect on the mouse vas deferens that the natural substance had.

The publication of the results from Hughes, Kosterlitz, and their colleagues was scheduled to be in the journal *Nature* of 18 December 1975. It reviewed the story so far: the opiate receptor discovery, and the sequence of events that had culminated in the discovery of enkephalin and the analysis of its structure. Pre-publication copies were sent off to friends and rivals. Solomon Snyder responded with a bottle of five-star cognac, a sporting gesture which did not go unappreciated by the British team.

But before the paper was even published, another British laboratory had become involved in the story, without their even knowing it. The point of contact was Howard Morris, who by this time had moved to Imperial College, in London. The occasion was a lecture, at Imperial College, by Derek Smyth of the National Institute for Medical Research.

Smyth and his group were looking for hormones secreted by the pituitary gland. Although the pituitary is at the base of the brain, just about the last thing Smyth was looking for was a chemical affecting the brain, since the pituitary's main job is to produce hormones to stimulate other glands in the body, such as the adrenals. Their main interest at the time was in a long peptide, containing more than ninety amino-acids, which seemed to contain a known hormone affecting the adrenals. There was also, at the tail of the molecule, a peptide already isolated by Dr Li, of San Francisco, whose action was quite unknown. To the astonishment of both Morris and Smyth, the first five amino-acids of this peptide were the familiar sequence of one of the forms of enkephalin: Tyr-Gly-Gly-Phe-Met. Howard Morris informed his colleagues, and Derek Smyth hurried back to the Institute to take a second look at his long peptide, which had so suddenly become important.

'We at once tested our peptides,' says Smyth, 'for binding to brain synaptosomes, and of course for the whole range of properties that morphine has, such as analgesia and effects on the blood pressure, and so on. Well . . . our peptide proves to be the most powerful naturally occuring analgesic agent that's been known. It proved to be a hundred times more potent than morphine.'

Since December 1975, when the Hughes, Kosterlitz et al., paper was published in *Nature*, research and publication on centrally acting peptides has turned from a trickle into a flood. The longer peptide has been given the name 'beta endorphin', and at least two variants have been identified, surrounded by the usual controversy. Enkephalin and beta endorphin (the word is a contraction of 'endogenous morphine') are commonly grouped together under the name endorphins, but also described as endogenous opiates. Derek Smyth would like to keep the name 'C fragment' for beta endorphin. Even the start of it all, enkephalin, comes in two varieties, one with the sequence of amino-acids ending with methionine, the other ending with leucine: they are described as met-enkephalin and leu-enkephalin, and have slightly different properties. The multiplicity of names perhaps reflects the multiple interpretations of their raison d'être and function.

At least some facts seem to be agreed. Enkephalin and beta endorphin are found in distinct, though largely different areas. Enkephalin is found in the brain, the spinal cord and the gut; beta endorphin in the brain, and apparently in the general circulation. The substances can actually be seen, glowing with an eerie light, in photographs where they have been stained with fluorescent dye, but because of the tiny amounts concerned they are still difficult to identify with absolute precision. They are relatively easy to synthesise, so large quantities are available for research.

As for the question of what they do, there is rather less agreement. Enkephalin only lasts for a few seconds in the body before it is broken down by enzymes, so it may qualify as a neurotransmitter, one of the chemicals which are used by brain cells to exchange signals; or maybe not. Beta-endorphin seems to last an hour or more before being broken down, and so does not seem to be a neurotransmitter; but what it could be described as is by no means clear.

What mysterious functions, then, do these 'keys of Paradise' unlock? One fairly clear activity they do seem to have is the control of pain, and it is in this field that much of the early research work was concentrated.

Dr Hosobuchi, at the University of California Medical School in San Francisco, has worked from early days in collaboration with Dr Li, who supplies the biochemical expertise and samples of the endorphins. Hosobuchi is a neurosurgeon, one of whose special skills is in the implantation of brain electrodes for the relief of pain, the sort of operation which Huda Akil did on her rats, but not, of course, this time for research purposes. Hosobuchi's patients are suffering from pain which cannot be relieved by any of the usual means.

The brain operation is a weird spectacle. The patient's head is clean-shaven and clamped into a framework so that it cannot move during the operation, in which Hosobuchi will have to locate a precise point in the brain. Because the patient has to report his or her sensations during the operation, he (or she) is also conscious throughout. Hosobuchi opens the skull with what looks like a superclean carpenter's brace and bit, and delicately inserts the electrodes into the patient's brain, watching his progress all the time on an X-ray machine. As he nears the appropriate place in the brain, he asks the patient to tell him what sensations are occuring, end eventually whether the pain has been abolished. By drawing off some of the fluid that normally bathes the brain, the cerebro-spinal fluid, Hosobuchi has established that, under the pain-abolishing electric stimulation, the amount of beta-endorphin in cerebro-spinal fluid has increased by up to eight times. Presumably this continues to be the case when the patient is equipped with his own electric stimulator for use when the operation is completed. The discovery certainly seems to confirm the connection between raised levels of beta-endorphin and abolition of pain.

Hosobuchi has done some more work which more directly suggests a pain-killing role for beta-endorphin. During the sort of operation already described, he has inserted tiny plastic reservoirs under the scalp, which feed beta-endorphin into the ventricles or cavities of the brain, so that it can enter the cerebro-spinal fluid. In these very few cases, which were done under the very strict rules relating to experiments on humans, it was clear that beta-endorphin did have an analgesic effect; but also that increasing doses were more effective, and that the effect was reversed by naloxone. So beta-endorphin does seem to operate through the opiate receptor system. The operation itself is so delicate that it is not likely to be available for normal patients; and beta-endorphin does not pass into the brain from the bloodstream, so is useless if it is injected intravenously.

The University of California Dental School has also played a part, but in an experiment far more controversial than Dr Hosobuchi's.

Howard Fields knew that anyone's perception of pain is to a great extent subjective, and dependent on the surroundings and situation of the sufferer. Soldiers in battle, for example, or football players during an important match, have been known to virtually ignore injuries, the pain of which would normally be incapacitating. In some proportion of cases it is possible to relieve pain which does not have an obvious cause, with a harmless, inert substance, a so-called placebo. Since a placebo is, essentially, an imaginary cure, doctors tend to assume that the pain it relieves is also imaginary. Fields decided to put some of these ideas to the test, in the context of what he had learned about endorphins.

The experiment he devised is at first sight tortuous, but in fact rather straightforward. Obviously Fields needed a real pain, inflicted in the normal course of events – which is where the Dental School came in. Extraction of a wisdom tooth rather reliably results in pain. Fields enlisted the help of the Dental School to put him in touch with patients who could be used as guinea-pigs without harm – except for feeling more pain, perhaps. Then he devised a double-blind experiment.

In a double-blind trial of this kind, neither the subject nor the experimenter knows which is the placebo and which the active drug. In Fields's plan the patients and the bottles of drugs (or placebos) were assigned numbers. Each patient, after the extraction of the wisdom tooth was given either a pain-killing drug or a placebo. One third of the patients had pain relief from the placebo. Then a second injection was given, this time of naloxone, which would abolish the effect of the drug; but would it also abolish the effect of the placebo?

(It says something for the scruples of the dental school personnel, incidentally, that they insisted that one in ten of the *second* injections should also be of a painkiller. Like the traditional firing squad, they did not know who gave the pain-causing shots!)

To Fields's delight, though not presumably to the delight of the dental patients, a significant number of those who had gained relief from the placebo reported that the relief was abolished by the naloxone injection. This strongly suggested that the endorphins were involved in the relief of pain, as Hosobuchi's work indicated.

But for Fields there was an equally important clinical lesson to be learned: 'I think many of us, myself included,' says Fields, 'felt that if a patient's pain was relieved by placebo, then the pain was of psychological origin, or was imaginary. In medicine, since we don't know very much, we have a tendency to use common sense a lot; and common sense says that if a pain is relieved by an imaginary cure, then the pain must be imaginary. I think that what our results indicate is that if the pain is relieved by placebo, then it's just as likely to be real, because we've now established a physiological basis for the placebo.'

In such a delicate area, results like these are controversial, and Fields knows it. 'I think the biggest resistance has been from people who have said, "Well, we all know the placebo simply means the patient's attitude has changed, and he's telling the doctor what the doctor wants to hear, but really his pain is the same." There is a group of people that has that attitude, and they simply do not believe these results.' Of course, reducing a psychological to a mere physiological explanation may appear to psychologists threatening, particularly as it indicates that in principle states very much up to now the domain of psychologists may be altered by chemical means. But many psychologists recognise that a physical description is an additional, rather than alternative, explanation.

There is still a huge gap between the discovery of enkephalin and endorphin, and a clear, convincing explanation of their function. It is an enormously fashionable field of research which must have the most rigorous standards applied to it if there is not to be a 'bandwagon effect': too many results from too many experiments, without a solid theoretical structure which can make sense of the data and allow real scientific progress. But the experiments already carried out, many of them by the pioneers, are too fascinating in their implications to ignore.

Huda Akil had a very personal reason for devising and taking part in one experiment: 'I was pregnant when beta-endorphin was discovered and characterised in the brain, and I felt that I was going through many psychological and physiological changes. I knew that hormones and neurotransmitters would have to be involved in them, and I wondered if beta-endorphin would not be one. And so it was a sort of merging of a personal life and a scientific life that led me to it.'

Akil started to take samples of her own blood, and of blood from other pregnant mothers; and the story turned out to be more complicated than she had expected. First, beta-endorphin levels in rat blood, from which most data came, are much higher than in human blood. This could be explained by the fact that rats possess a small extra lobe in the pituitary gland (which secretes beta-endorphin); this extra lobe is very rich in beta-endorphin. Very oddly, it is present in human foetuses, and is thought to reappear in the mother during pregnancy; and Akil found a much higher than normal content of beta-endorphin in blood during pregnancy and labour, and also a high content in blood from the umbilical cords of children born during the survey. Why? What is it doing?

'All I can say is that Nature does not do these things trivially. I would not be happy guessing too fast, particularly because we don't know what blood beta-endorphin does. We don't know where it's going, we don't know what it's trying to affect, we don't know whether it gets to the baby, or whether the baby's stuff gets to the mother. So there are too many questions to speculate, but it's interesting enough to hang on to, and keep doing more with it.'

One hypothesis which has gained a number of adherents is

that endorphins modulate, or at least play a part in, our perception of pleasure as well as of pain. To put this another way, there is a continuum of reward, at the lower end of which is pain (the opposite of reward) and at the upper end the sort of satisfaction which accompanies eating, sexual gratification, and possibly reflects the sort of needs exemplified in drug addiction or alcoholism. Experiments have been done to establish levels of endorphins in the circulation of obese patients who appear to be compulsive eaters; and to link endorphin levels with sexual behaviour in hamsters. This sort of connection remains to be firmly established, but Candace Pert probably speaks for many researchers when she says, 'Maybe God put the vas deferens there for John Hughes to discover enkephalin, but somehow I doubt it. I have a feeling it has to be a sexual role. That's a speculation, and it's the hypothesis we're currently examining.'

Floyd Bloom, at the Salk Institute near San Diego in Southern California, has done some work with alcoholic rats which leads him to 'propose, then, as a working hypothesis that the enjoyable part as your blood alcohol is going up – that kind of vivacious, improved spirituality-attitude that one has during that early stage of a cocktail party – that might be an endorphin-like effect.'

But Bloom has done much more work on the new peptides, much of it initially with Roger Guillemin, who won a Nobel Prize for isolating and establishing the structure of some of the hormones released by the brain. Bloom and Guillemin were both interested to see what effect endorphins might have on the behaviour of animals – specifically the laboratory rat. Said Bloom, 'Every new substance that's extracted from the brain goes through a sort of natural history where people finally isolate and characterise the molecule, and then, not knowing where in the brain it might work, we take the very bold step of putting it some place in the brain that can get to every place in the brain. Usually something not very pronounced will happen.' That was not the case with beta-endorphin.

Bloom and his colleagues fitted up one of their laboratory rats with an electro-encephalogram apparatus, which shows the electrical activity of the brain, this time in the form of pen traces on a moving strip of paper. Then they infused a dose of beta-endorphin into the animal's brain. Outwardly, the rat showed very little change in its behaviour. But, says Bloom, 'We were totally amazed. The animal was doing absolutely nothing and yet there was his head absolutely generating an entire village's worth of electricity, it appeared to be, and the pens – they were raking right off the paper, ink splattering everywhere ... with the animal's sole behaviour an occasional wet-dog shake and then sniffing the air ... and then lapsing into this vacant stare, followed by the extreme rigidity and the total unresponsiveness to painful stimuli.'

After their first astonishment, Bloom and Guillemin realised that the vacant stare and rigidity of the rat reminded them of catatonic patients whom they had seen in early days of medical training. They had what seemed, says Bloom, 'a harebrained idea'. Catatonia was a fairly frequent symptom of some forms of schizophrenia. Rigidity in the rats was swiftly abolished by naloxone; so would naloxone relieve at least some of the symptoms of schizophrenia? Until Guillemin attended a conference in Europe, they had no idea that the same idea had occurred to the ubiquitous Lars Terenius.

Terenius had established, to his own satisfaction, that cerebro-spinal fluid from schizophrenic patients often showed raised endorphin levels. With the help of a psychiatrist, Lief Lindstrom, six schizophrenic patients with auditory hallucinations were given naloxone. Four of the six reported that the sounds in their head stopped. Similar experiments in the United States appeared to be successful too, but many less successful attempts were made, and many doctors reported that naloxone did not help. 'I think,' says Terenius, 'that schizophrenia can derive from a number of different disorders or defects of the nervous system. If you have a flat tyre, you can't drive the car, but it can be any one of the tyres. It's the same with schizophrenia: it can be due to one of several different systems.' So at present it appears that the case for treating schizophrenic patients with naloxone is at best not proven. But that is not to say that endorphins are unconnected with the condition, and further research may turn up clearer connections.

Perhaps the most exciting of all the effects that have been seen is to do with learning and memory. More than one group has reported that very small doses of endorphin given to rats subcutaneously seem to improve learning capacity. This seems extraordinary, since the dose cannot pass the blood-brain barrier, and thus cannot reach the brain. It goes without saying that there is a vast difference between rats and humans, and that what psychologists call learning, in rats, is a very different matter, in degree at least, from human memory. But the work does have very significant implications. Lars Terenius: 'It's one of the big problems in our civilisation that we can keep people organically alive, but not mentally alive. In maybe ten or fifteen years from now, senility is probably going to be the big problem for medical research. It is also possible that some of these peptides can be used to improve the retrieval of memory previously stored within the brain.'

The story began with an attempt to discover the causes of drug addiction. Sadly, it has not so far led to that discovery or to any new treatment for addiction. However, it does seem possible that morphine and heroin addicts are suffering from an inherent biochemical imbalance; if so, they are organically ill, and not suffering from some moral incapacity such as lack of will-power.

The fact is, the biochemistry of the brain is far, far more complex than we yet understand. The discovery of the endorphins shows it to be more complex than we imagined ten years ago, and more discoveries will complicate the picture still further. But each new discovery also adds to our sum of knowledge, and eventually this collection of facts will take shape. It takes many man-years of scientific effort to establish even one small fact beyond dispute; and however much we may speculate on the implications, those speculations have to be tested and proved before we can make proper use of them. There may even be dangers; a little learning is a dangerous thing.

There is probably no area of science more important than our understanding of ourselves, which must mean to a great degree, our understanding of how our brains work. If we can learn enough about the biochemistry of our brains, it is possible that we shall be able to make drugs to correct mistakes in the functioning of the brain: something to help old people remember better, as Terenius suggested, for example.

As soon as Hughes and Kosterlitz announced the discovery of the first opiate peptide, enkephalin, the drug companies began research at a furious pace to find a way of making drugs which would relieve pain as well as morphine, but without its harmful side-effects. There were considerable problems to overcome. Enkephalin breaks down so quickly that it is quite useless as a drug; beta-endorphin will not cross the blood-brain barrier. By rearranging the molecules, substituting different amino-acids for the natural ones, the pharmaceutical firms have overcome both of these problems, but have not yet succeeded in producing the safe, powerful analgesic for which they had hoped. One that did look promising as a pain-killer also turned out to partly paralyse the legs. Other compounds had other problems, underlining the complexity of the system. It may be more fruitful to find a drug which will stop the natural breakdown of the endorphins, rather than finding substitutes for them. It may take some years before there is a useful drug based on the discoveries of 1975, but it will almost certainly happen – eventually.

In a way, the story of 'The Keys of Paradise' has no ending. But it does exemplify an era in which it became clear, for everyone working in those sciences which examine the profound mysteries of the human brain, that there were many new discoveries around the corner. Since 1975, numbers of other substances have been isolated and identified; and receptors have been found for the benzodiazepine group of tranquillisers which includes Valium and Librium. The techniques which have been developed will make further discoveries easier; but perhaps nothing in the future will have quite the same impact on those people who were part of the story.

Perhaps the best summing-up comes from Huda Akil: 'I think it's very rare that a scientist is privileged to watch the birth of a new era, if you will, in his or her field. It was something like wating for the sun to come out, and all of a sudden it does. It had that feeling about it. We knew it was there, we knew it was important, but nobody could quite get a hold on it – and then all of a sudden there it was in your lap. And I remember thinking, "I'm never going to forget these days, because I may never live through anything like this ever again." '

One of the first results of the introduction of the transatlantic telegraph was the catching of a criminal. Today it is quite normal for detectives (including medical ones) to obtain information from other parts of the world – particularly the Western world – through telexes, telephones, satellites and computer terminals. The work on endorphins and other brain chemicals was, and is, very much an international affair. Long gone are the days when discoveries are made by a Pasteur or a Fleming working virtually alone. Even the discovery of the double helix in DNA in the 1950s was a race between groups who knew very well what the other groups, in other countries, were doing.

In one particular field of medicine, it was realised that the necessary clues would not be forthcoming without a fairly complicated inter-national computer network. That was the field of immunology and in particular the work on antigens, part of the body's defence system. If DNA contains the blueprints for making cells, then antigens are the fingerprints of each type of cell. Fingerprints, blueprints and blood – all the ingredients for another international thriller! In the same way that fingerprints are passed around between police forces, the information about blood cells was to be passed rapidly between different research groups all round the world.

5 Blueprints in the Bloodstream

Vivienne King

Every living being, from man to mouse, is uniquely different from every other, even at the microscopic level of its cells. Not only that, but every living being has evolved a complex system for distinguishing foreign from self. It is this system which makes the body recognise a transplant as foreign – and reject it; or spot invading bacteria – and attack them. The key lies in a set of microscopic fingerprints on the surface of our cells. White cells in the bloodstream, called leucocytes, fight off the continuous assault of viruses and bacteria. In this invisible defensive force are several different categories of cell. Among them are the T-cells, which carry out a continuous surveillance operation. They patrol blood vessels and tissue, on the look-out for foreign organisms. These foreign organisms are given away by a system of markers called antigens on the surfaces of their cells: these are also a kind of molecular fingerprint, different from the body's own.

Some T-cells react to foreign antigens by a direct attack on the hostile organism. Others react by spreading the alarm to the lymph glands, home of the next line of defence: the B-cells. These cells are chemical factories for making antibody. Once alerted, they swarm to the site of infection, releasing molecules of antibody like chemical bullets. These molecules fasten onto the foreign antigens providing a toehold which allows the body's scavenger cells to dispose of them. It is a system that has been understood in principle, if not in detail, since 1885.

In 1980 Professor Jean Dausset, now working at the Hospital St Louis in Paris, was awarded the Nobel Prize for medicine for his pioneering work in a branch of immunology which has revolutionised transplant surgery. But its major impact could be in a quite separate area – in the field of preventive medicine. It could explain why some of us fight off certain diseases, while others succumb. Already, it has thrown new light on a number of mysterious illnesses, including diabetes, rheumatoid arthritis and multiple sclerosis. Ultimately it could lead to their prevention.

This extraordinary story has its origins in an unlikely setting: the battlefields of France. During the Second World War, Dausset was a field doctor in the army. He noticed that his patients sometimes had a violent reaction to blood transfusions, although their blood groups had been correctly matched. At this stage, nobody knew why.

After the war, Dausset returned to his work in Paris, studying diseases of the blood, and in 1952 he made another observation. Down the microscope he saw a battle going on in a sample of a patient's blood. But the patient's immune defence system was attacking a *human* cell. It was mounting a massive antibody attack on a white blood cell, exactly as if it was a virus or a bacterium. This had never been seen before.

Publication of this bizarre phenomenon set off a train of events around the world. At Stanford University, Rose Payne looked for, and found, the same phenomenon in one of her own patients. She wondered if this explained the victim's low white-cell count. Was his body attacking his own cells? Then she realised that the white cell under attack was not the patient's own. It had got there as the result of a blood transfusion.

All these patients had one thing in common. They had received, not one, but several blood transfusions. When patients reacted to a blood transfusion, they were reacting, not to the red cells, which had been correctly matched, but to foreign *white* cells in the transfusion brew. At the first transfusion, nothing happens. But the patient's immune response system has nevertheless been alerted, and it has formed antibodies to the foreign cells. At the next transfusion, the body is primed to react; and it mounts a massive antibody attack. This reaction produces symptoms of high fever and chills, like a bad attack of flu as the body reacts to the system of antigens on the surface of the donor's white blood cells. Dausset was the first to realise that white cells carry these markers. It meant that each individual has two sorts of blood group: the familiar red cell group, A, B, O or AB, and a second, white cell type. His chance discovery was to have repercussions far beyond the walls of the blood banks: it was to reach into all branches of medicine.

But first, there was the problem of how to classify a patient's white cell type. Red cell typing is relatively simple, since there are only four blood groups. But white cell typing turned out to be much more complex, for there are many, many more types. And each one of us has, not one, but at least eight different types of antigen on the surface of our cells. They are impossible to see even under the microscope, so you are 'typed' according to the antibodies your white cells react with. To do this, scientists needed a ready source of human antibody in large amounts. But from where?

This problem was solved unexpectedly in Holland, in the blood bank of a Leiden hospital. Jan Van Rood was one day called to the bedside of a young mother who had just given birth to twins. She had reacted violently to a blood transfusion following the delivery. Van Rood was familiar with the symptoms – he'd seen them before in multiple-transfusion patients. He took a sample and found there were, indeed, antibodies to human cells circulating in her blood. But this woman had never received a blood transfusion before in her life. So how had they got there?

Light dawned. The mother had formed antibodies against her babies. A child developing in the womb represents a massive invasion of the mother's body by foreign cells. As the baby grows, its cells divide and die. Dead cells from the foetus pass through the placenta – and into the mother's bloodstream. Half the antigens on these cells will be like hers. But the other half are inherited from the baby's father – and therefore alien. Once in the mother's bloodstream, these foreign antigens will be spotted by T-cells, and she will make antibodies to them. This happens in about a third of all pregnancies. The antibody does not reach the baby, so it does no harm. But it remains circulating in the mother's blood for ten or twenty years, and can prime her body for an attack on alien cells in a blood transfusion.

Events in Leiden provided a kind of scientific launch-pad for research. Van Rood had found in many human mothers a treasure trove of human antibodies – molecular keys for detecting the antigens on our own white cells. Mix a patient's cells with a set of antibodies, and you get a set of reactions. The white cell type could be classified according to these reactions. But how should the classification be organised? In 1961, British geneticist Walter Bodmer and his wife Julia were on sabbatical at Stanford University in California. Here they met Rose Payne. She explained her problem: how could these complex sets of reactions be organised into groups, like the red cell blood groups? It was a problem in statistics. Julia wrote a programme, and the first cell types emerged from the computer, starkly named A1 and A2. It was one of the first applications of computer techniques in medicine.

After that, research took off across the world with un-precedented speed. Scientists collaborated in a unique global experiment. They met regularly for international workshops at which results were pooled and collated. Soon, they had typed the world. They had data from every continent except Antarctica. They called the system HLA: human leucocyte antigens. Molecular fingerprints on the surface of human cells, they spelt out an individual's biochemical identity.

We inherit our HLA type from our parents, exactly as we inherit the colour of our hair and eyes. The genes which code for them are all located on a single chromosome, Chromosome 6. In the Sixties, two distinct groups of antigens were identified, though more have been discovered since. Each individual is classified by two A-types and two B-types – one from each parent. For example (A1 B8), (A2 B12). The number of different A and B types is enormous. Over twenty of each have been found, though they are not all to be found in any one single race: for example, the Australian Aboriginals do not have B27. There are millions of possible combinations, so there's not much chance of two people sharing exactly the same type, unless they are brothers and sisters: then the chance is one in four. Even at the level of our cells, we are all different from each other.

Family Tree 1

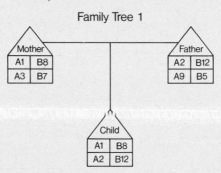

Pattern of inheritance of HLA types. The child has inherited types (A1 B8) from its mother and types (A2 B12) from its father.

As data poured out around the world, a fresh thought struck researchers. If the HLA type provided a key to biological uniqueness, could it also be the key to why patients reject skin grafts or organ transplants from other donors? And so, in the mid-Sixties, scientists began a bizarre series of experiments with skin grafts, first among themselves, and then with volunteers. They swopped tiny pieces of skin, about as large as a new penny.

Generally the graft would last for about ten days. Then it would slough off, rejected. HLA researchers travelled around the world, accumulating strings of little circular scars on their fore-arms, living proof of the body's effective rejection process. But as they had hoped, it turned out that these grafts lasted better if A and B types were matched.

So white cell types were in fact tissue types: they classified human tissue. Indeed, these same antigens were to be found on almost every cell in the human body, except the red blood cells. The HLA system comes into play whenever the body is invaded by foreign tissue: for example, white cells in blood transfusions, the foetus in a pregnant mother; and, of course, transplanted organs.

Tissue-typing is now a powerful weapon in the transplant surgeon's armoury. When a kidney becomes available, the immediate problem is to find a recipient with matching A and B types. But because they vary so enormously, it's hard to find a perfect match. And in transplant surgery, time is short. It may be only a matter of hours before the kidney cells die. So a worldwide network has been set up. In Leiden, Van Rood set up Euro-transplant. In Britain, the UK Transplant Service is based in Bristol. These centres hold computerised records of kidney patients. Through a fast data-link system it is possible to match kidney to patient in a matter of hours. HLA typing has also proved valuable for bone-marrow transplants and for corneal grafting. In heart transplants it is less useful. Hearts are less available, and the organ goes to whoever can use it, regardless of type. The problem of rejection is dealt with by damping down the patient's immune response – making him tragically vulner-able to infections.

By the end of the Sixties, HLA typing had transformed pros-pects for patients undergoing transplant surgery. It had opened up research into other, more exotic possibilities, such as trans-planting healthy pancreas tissue into diabetics. It had revolution-ised a whole area of medicine, albeit at the high-cost/high-technology end of the market. But one fundamental question remained unanswered. Why should HLA be there? The system could hardly have been devised by a teasing Creator simply to torment transplant surgeons.

Clues came from work on lowlier creatures. It had long been known that mice possess an equivalent system of tissue-types, called H2. It controls the survival of grafts between animals. This had been studied by scientists like George Snell and Baruj

Benacerref in the USA, who were jointly to share the 1980 Nobel Prize with Jean Dausset. But in 1964 in New York, scientist Frank Lilly noticed that mice with a certain tissue-type were especially vulnerable to a form of leukaemia caused by a virus. If they had that type, they died when exposed to the virus. If not, they survived.

Was HLA linked with human disease? For years, they searched in vain for a connection. It turned up unexpectedly in 1971, at the Westminster Hospital in London; not with leukaemia, but with a painful form of rheumatism.

Doctors had begun to suspect that rheumatic disorders could be caused by defects in the immune response; and rheumatism runs in families. So at the Westminster Hospital, they decided to check the tissue-types of all their patients. It seemed a long shot – but to their astonishment, they found an extremely strong connection with an unpleasant form of rheumatism called ankylosing spondylitis. Over ninety per cent of patients shared a common tissue-type – B27.

Ankylosing spondylitis is hardly a household name. It's one of those rare and baffling diseases, hard to treat, and often hard to diagnose. In its severest form it causes 'poker spine', a complete fusing together of the vertebrae, usually leaving the sufferer in a rigidly bent-over position. One patient complained he was afraid to cross the road, because he couldn't stand up to look out for traffic. In women, this degeneration of the bones is harder to spot, though the pain is real enough. Late diagnosis makes treatment even harder, and many female patients suffer from accusations of neurosis, hysteria – or simply lead-swinging.

Ankylosing spondylitis seemed to run in families, though the inheritance pattern was not clear. But when the B27 connection turned up, it provided doctors with a genetic handle for understanding the disease. Only seven per cent of the British population has the B27 tissue-type, so this might explain the rarity of the disease.

In Los Angeles, Paul Terasaki confirmed the Westminster findings. He studied different racial groups in the local community. 'In Japan,' says Terasaki, 'the B27 antigen is almost non-existent; very few people have it. And yet essentially all the patients that have ankylosing spondylitis, that are Japanese, have the B27 antigen. We looked at some Negroes and found that even there, even though the disease is rare, patients that have ankylosing spondylitis tend to have B27.'

At Westminster, rheumatologists had noticed a puzzling

assortment of symptoms associated with the disease, though not necessarily complications of it. For example, psoriasis, a skin complaint, ulcerative colitis, a disease of the gut, and iritis, a painful inflammation of the eye, any of these may be around if there is ankylosing spondylitis. These conditions also seemed to run in families, in various combinations. For example, take the Kennedy family from London. Mrs Kennedy and her sister both have ankylosing spondylitis. Her daughter Jennifer has psoriasis – but not spondylitis. Her daughter Lynne doesn't have psoriasis – but she has iritis, and arthritis in her joints.

Dr Derek Brewerton, consultant rheumatologist at Westminster hospital, wondered if tissue-typing patients like these would throw any light on the situation: 'We knew that a third of patients with ankylosing spondylitis may develop iritis, an acute inflammation of the eyes. And yet most patients who have iritis don't have ankylosing spondylitis at all. And it doesn't really behave like a complication. So we wondered whether the connection between the two disorders might be inherited; in which case, if we looked at people who had iritis without any rheumatic disease at all, then we might find a marker there.'

Moorfields Eye Hospital sent him a hundred patients as they turned up at their casualty eye clinic. And true enough, over forty per cent of the patients with acute iritis, *without* rheumatic disease, had the same marker, B27. This meant that a Londoner born with B27 was twenty times as likely to end up at Moorfields with iritis as the rest of the population.

So patients who were B27 positive had somehow inherited a kind of vulnerability to all these diseases. They might acquire some or all of the symptoms during their lives – or alternatively, none. With many inherited diseases, the genetic connection is simple. If you're born with the gene for haemophilia, you'll be a haemophiliac. But people who inherit the B27 gene and tissue-type do not simply inherit a disease – they inherit a *susceptibility*. Some other factor in their environment must trigger off the disease. What kind of trigger factor? Evidence came from another unexpected source: a report by a ship's doctor on the US Navy's *Little Rock*.

On 2 June 1962 this ship had docked at Trieste. 1200 marines went ashore, among them the two chefs. Unfortunately for him, but fortunately for the progress of medical science, one of the chefs caught a nasty dose of shigella dysentery. Later, he helped prepare a barbecue – and spread dysentery among 600 of the crew. Four weeks later, ten of these ill-fated crew-members developed Reiter's disease, a painful and crippling form of arthritis, so severely that they were invalided out. The ship's doctor dutifully wrote up his report.

In 1973, Dr Andrei Calin happened to read this strange account. It struck him as a marvellous natural experiment. The ship was a perfect floating laboratory: ten neat case-studies for a tissue-typing sleuth. Locating them was quite a problem, because of the reluctance of the Naval Authorities to release such highly confidential information. But eventually he managed to track down five of the victims, and found to his delight that four of them were B27 positive.

It had long been known that Reiter's syndrome could be triggered off by bacterial gut infections, like yersinia, shigella, or salmonella; or non-specific urethritis, a venereal infection. Calin's work revealed that a patient with B27 is forty times more likely than the rest of us to develop arthritis after such an infection, regardless of whether the initial infection ever produces symptoms.

These findings turned the world of rheumatology upside down. It was a major breakthrough in a baffling field of medicine: the first really strong result in decades of fruitless research. It seems that certain genes in the HLA system increase our chances of developing rheumatism and arthritis. In other words, we may inherit a susceptibility to those diseases. But the symptoms have to be triggered off by something in the environment – probably a virus or bacterium. If doctors could isolate that trigger, it might be possible to vaccinate those at risk – perhaps even, one day, to eliminate the diseases.

Following the rheumatologists' breakthrough came more exciting evidence. Doctors began to conjecture that when we become ill, it is not through pure chance. It could be that, from birth, we are susceptible to certain diseases. These weaknesses may be programmed in our genes. Even the course of those diseases, the symptoms we get, or the way we respond to drug treatment, may be a consequence of the genes we carry on Chromosome 6. For it is not only rheumatism that is implicated.

The next disease to be investigated by tissue-typers was diabetes, in which patients lose their natural control of blood sugar levels. Some survive by taking tablets and watching their diets. But for many more it means daily injections of insulin, without which they would die. Sometimes, the disease begins in middle age. Tragically, it often strikes the very young.

Through the discovery of insulin thousands of patients had been saved, and the disease had been brought under control; but it remained something of a mystery. Again, it runs in families, though the inheritance pattern wasn't clear. Children of diabetics do not inevitably acquire the disease. And diabetic children may have perfectly healthy parents. Again, there was anecdotal evidence that a virus might be involved. There were reports of outbreaks following mumps epidemics; other surveys implicated the coxsackie virus. High levels of antibodies to these two viral infections had been found in patients' blood serum soon after onset of diabetes. And most cases of diabetes seemed to occur in winter, suggesting a winter virus. Further, there was the observation that the childhood disease peaks at the ages of five and eleven, when children are either starting or changing schools. New environments, new viruses.

In 1974, Andrew Cudworth, a Liverpool doctor, read about ankylosing spondylitis and the B27 connection. He wondered whether tissue-typing could create any kind of order in the chaos of diabetic research. He began a survey in the Liverpool area, later extended to the rest of Britain, and repeated throughout the world. What emerged was a strong correlation with HLA type B8.

From it, one important new factor could be deduced. It was clear from the tissue-typing studies that 'diabetes' was not one single disease, but two. The middle-age onset type is quite distinct, and probably due to nutritional factors. It is inherited,

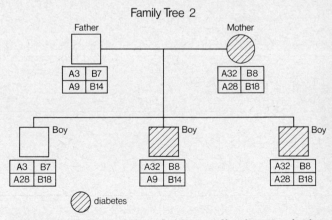

Family Tree 2

In this family the mother has diabetes. So have two of her three sons: they have also inherited from her the B8 gene.

but not through the B8 gene. The HLA connection was with juvenile-onset diabetes, always more serious, always insulin-dependent. The pattern of inheritance showed up clearly in Cudworth's family trees. But again, there had to be an environmental trigger – further evidence for the virus connection.

HLA typing had not yielded all the answers, but it set research off in a new direction. During the Seventies, almost every disease was checked for tissue-type connections. More and more previously baffling diseases became implicated: coeliac disease (a disease of the gut), chronic auto-immune hepatitis (a disease of the liver), myasthenia gravis (a wasting disease of muscle and nerve), Graves' disease (a disease of the thyroid gland), Addison's disease (a type of anaemia), dermatitis herpetiformis (a skin disease), paralytic poliomyelitis – even psychiatric illnesses like schizophrenia and manic depression. And there are many more.

Not only does our HLA type control the diseases we acquire, but it even influences the course they take. For example, a chronic alcoholic who is B8 positive is much more likely to develop cirrhosis of the liver. So perhaps what every drinker needs to know above all is his tissue type! As Rose Payne puts it, these markers on our cells are 'beacon lights of susceptibility'. The genetic dice are loaded, from before birth.

As things stood in the mid-Seventies, research results were exciting – but of mainly academic interest. The disease associations were offering a tantalising glimpse into future patterns of medicine, yet they were not strong enough to provide any further breakthroughs. Compared with the B27 connections, many of the associations were relatively weak. They were there, but in as few as thirty or forty per cent of patients. Scientists suspected the genes for the A and B types were being inherited in tandem with others, on the same chromosome, which could provide a stronger link. They had already found a third, C type. But it was not involved in these diseases. The A and B types were clearly part of the system which alerts the body to invasion by foreign tissue – probably also to infection by viruses and bacteria. But there might be a fourth type directly controlling the immune response. In mice, these genes had already been found. They were called 'I_R' genes. They switch the immune response on or off – and control how high or low that response may be. In man, such genes had not been found.

The next significant milestone in the HLA story was reached in Van Rood's laboratory. It arose from those bizarre experiments with skin grafts. He was experimenting with ways and means of keeping those tiny transplants going. 'Every day we won, if we could apply that to kidney grafting, it would mean that the kidney graft would survive, not one day, but one year longer. You see, in this game, every day counts.' One of his volunteers was a Mrs Plug. 'We thought we had fixed things in a certain way that the skin graft should slough off after, say, between twelve and fourteen days. But at fourteen days she was fine and at fifteen and sixteen, and so on. And only when it was twenty-two days the skin graft sloughed off. And we could not understand it with the information we had at that time.'

Mrs Plug had been given a skin graft which did not match her A and B type. Yet somehow it had survived. She had been accidentally matched for a new HLA type – a fourth, D type of antigen. These antigens had been missed because they are only to be found on certain leucocytes – on the B cells which make antibody.

Scientists now had a more complete picture of the genes in this vital region of Chromosome 6. Were the new D-types the missing genes? Did they directly control the immune response, like the I_R genes in the mouse? Scientists are still not sure. It seems likely. But if not, they are very close to the ones which do. For the D-types turned out to be of paramount importance in transplant work. If D-types are matched, the chances of success are orders of magnitude higher – even if A and B types differ. In bone-marrow transplants, D-type matching is critical to success or failure.

The discovery of the new types offered further help for transplant surgeons. For if the D-types are the key to why a transplant is rejected, doctors might prolong survival by 'fine-tuning' the patient's immune response. Instead of blocking the entire system with immuno-suppressive drugs, effectively 'blindfolding' the body's surveillance system, they might find ways of sealing off only the D-antigen response. In rats it's already possible. Such fine-tuning might transform prospects for heart transplant patients.

As for disease associations, the D-types proved to be much more powerful markers, drawing more diseases into the net. For example, doctors had been unable to find an HLA association with rheumatoid arthritis – surprising in view of the other B27 connections. Now they found a strong correlation with HLA D4. But most revealing of all, the D-types were especially strongly connected with diseases where the immune response goes wild and attacks the patient's own tissue – diseases like multiple sclerosis.

MS is one of the most puzzling and tragic diseases of the developed world in the twentieth century – a disease in which patients mistake their own tissue for something foreign. Their white cells attack the protective sheath around nerves in the brain and spinal cord, destroying connections and causing weird visual distortions and increasing paralysis.

There are weak family patterns. Perhaps one in ten patients has a relative who is also affected. And again, worldwide research has led to the conclusion that there is some environmental trigger. Almost everything has been blamed – from climate to animal fat to measles.

At the peak of the HLA euphoria, doctors began tissue-typing MS patients. Any new research handle was worth a try. But results were disappointing. Thirty per cent had the A3 type; forty per cent had B7. It wasn't very significant. Then came the D-types, and researchers began to feel they were getting closer. Sixty per cent of patients were D2 positive. But it still wasn't as good as they'd hoped. Then yet another new HLA type was identified – once again, on B-cells only. At the Royal Victoria Hospital in East Grinstead, Richard Batchelor devised a test for detecting this fifth type. And with a colleague, neurologist Dr Alistair Compston, he began retesting MS patients. Eighty per cent of them shared the same type – now called DR2.

After years of fruitless and often contradictory research, it was the first strong lead ever to emerge. With this new knowledge, they were able to identify a high-risk group. Long-term studies over many years of DR2-positive people, both healthy and sick, could establish how this tragic disease develops – and find the trigger.

Already, the HLA connection has fitted one piece into the jig-saw. The course of MS varies considerably in different patients, making the disease hard to diagnose. Some patients have one attack, recover, and never have another. Others get progressively worse, until they are almost totally paralysed. But the first symptom is often optic neuritis – a bizarre disturbance of vision, in which patients may see double, or temporarily lose their sight. However, patients with optic neuritis do not inevitably develop MS.

Alastair Compston and Professor Ian McDonald carried out a trial at London's National Hospital for Nervous Diseases. They searched the records for patients who had presented with optic neuritis, thirty years ago; they traced them, and tissue-typed them. Some now had MS, others didn't. But over ninety per cent of those who *had* developed MS were DR2 positive. So patients with optic neuritis who also have the DR2 type are nearly fifty times as likely to develop MS as the rest of the population. Furthermore, of those who now had MS, most had developed their visual symptoms in the winter: strong, though not conclusive evidence for a winter virus.

Through such long-term studies of high-risk groups, doctors hope to build up a profile of this mystifying disease. They may ultimately discover what triggers off MS in the susceptible. They may even discover why it is that some drugs help certain patients, but not others. For many of these drugs work through their effect on the immune response. In MS patients, this is faulty – and the key to these individual characteristics, how the patients react to infections and to such drugs, could lie in the HLA type. In modern drug trials, it is now always taken into account.

Most of this HLA research is at present of value only to other researchers. It has produced no magic cures. But some of it could be applied now: in Third World countries, the benefits could be immediate. For recently it has been found that HLA is associated with leprosy. This disease is still endemic in much of the world. It can be prevented, but the protective drug is expensive, and the side effects are painful. To treat the entire population of India or the Sudan would be inconceivable. But leprosy does run in families. By tissue-typing them, doctors could identify high-risk children, and vaccinate only them with the precious drugs.

Meanwhile, the list of disease associations continues to grow. In Copenhagen, Arne Svejgaard keeps the tally. Data from every corner of the globe is stored in his computer. He is building up a world picture of disease. Now that infectious diseases like cholera and TB are under control, the diseases which correlate so strongly with the HLA system are going to be more important. At first, cancer seemed to be excluded. Now a connection has been found with one rare form. But even without cancer, we are probably talking about fifty per cent or more of the diseases we are most likely to get.

So long is the list that the very number of diseases involved seems to cast doubt on the veracity of it all. Some are immune response diseases, such as coeliac disease or MS. Others are hormonal, such as juvenile-onset diabetes. Myasthenia gravis is a quite different illness, in which signals from nerve endings are somehow blocked, and are not received in the connecting muscle. And then there are the psychiatric illnesses, like schizophrenia. How could HLA possibly be involved in all these?

There are several theories.

1 'Molecular mimicry'
A virus may gain foothold in the body by mimicry. Usually, a viral intruder is given away by the antigen markers on its surface. But what if these markers look like our own? For example, suppose the virus causing ankylosing spondylitis looks like the B27 antigen. Then patrolling T-cells in a B27 patient may be fooled, and fail to mount an immune attack.

2 'Altered self'
Once a virus has lodged itself in a human cell, it may tamper with machinery in the nucleus and actually alter the antigens on the cell's surface. So the patient's own cells change identity, and look foreign. The body then attacks them.

3 'Receptor confusion'
HLA antigens act as receptor sites on the surfaces of our cells. It's possible that they may closely resemble other receptor sites on the same cell – for example, hormone receptor sites. If so, hormones could mistakenly 'lock in' to the wrong receptor, and fail to transmit their chemical message to the cell.

This could explain the HLA association with so-called 'endocrine' or hormonal diseases. In psychiatric illness there might be a similar mechanism. HLA receptor sites might interfere with the chemical messages between neurones in the brain. And in myasthenia gravis, the HLA receptor sites might block the transmission of nerve impulses from nerve-ending to muscle.

HLA research has opened up whole new gateways into our understanding of diseases. But how will it actually help the sick? The implications could be controversial. For example, it is now possible to tissue-type an unborn baby. But would we abort the foetus at risk of diabetes or multiple sclerosis?

A suggestion comes from Jean Dausset. HLA markers are carried by sperm. A baby's future is to some extent determined at the moment of conception – when the sperm strikes the egg. If the sperm which carry markers for certain diseases could be eliminated, then artificial insemination with 'safe' sperm would ensure the baby's future. Science fiction? In veterinary practice, it's already possible.

As medicine looks to the future through HLA, geneticists look to the past, struggling to understand how the system has evolved. They believe it could be one of the oldest gene systems, dating right back to the beginnings of evolution. Systems like HLA are found in almost all animals – in toads, in reptiles and in birds. Take two worms from different gardens and cut them in half: the two 'foreign' halves will not join up: 'matched' ones, from the same garden, will. Swim down to a coral reef: one type of coral will never grow on another.

While HLA may have played a key role in our early development, in the course of evolution it has also been crucial to our survival. The enormous variety of HLA, more diverse than any other gene system yet discovered, could have been crucial to the continuing survival of the human species, in defending us against centuries of plagues and epidemics. Exceptional in this diversity are the Red Indians, whose HLA types are very limited. This could explain why they were almost wiped out by European diseases.

Ironically, these very genes which have guaranteed survival through cholera, TB, plague and earlier ravages, now seem to make us vulnerable – to degenerative diseases like rheumatoid arthritis, or the diseases of modern Western affluence, like multiple sclerosis and diabetes. Now, it is up to man's ingenuity to use his new knowledge of himself through HLA to conquer these diseases.

A fundamental characteristic of scientific research is the return to basics. It always seems to be going backwards, to search for evolution and origins. (In this sense it parts company from the detective's work which seldom has to look for common elements in large numbers of crimes or criminals). Only by going back to basics can the investigators build a framework of theory to help them go forward.

In physics, all work now centres around sub-atomic particles. In medicine, that basis is genetics. The decoding of genes is the fundamental activity. In the same way that every physical phenomenon can be expressed in terms of the energy associated with particle interaction, so genes 'express' every medical phenomenon. Research into interferon, brown fat cells, brain chemicals, and HLA, all involve gene expression. But there is one fundamental and clearly obvious result of differences in gene expression – the differences in sex.

6 The Fight to be Male

Edward Goldwyn

Where does masculinity and femininity come from? Is our sexual behaviour deeply part of us when we are born or do we learn to be our sex? Research over the last few years has sharpened these questions. There have been quite unexpected insights into the details of how a human egg will develop to become a male or female baby. This has thrown light on the differences in behaviour of the sexes – of the masculine, the feminine and the in-betweens.

Back in the 1950s, Professor Alfred Jost startled the scientific community by showing that the natural form of the human is the female; a male is the result of interference with 'natural' foetal development. It had been known for decades that it is the sperm, from the male, which decides the sex of a fertilised egg. The egg carries an X chromosome, the sperm either an X or a Y. If the fertilisation is by an X-bearing sperm the XX egg develops to a female. If the sperm is a Y-bearing, the XY egg develops to a male. It was while unravelling the process of how that development took place that Jost made his pronouncement. The steps of this process as currently understood are these:

First, female development. The egg is fertilised by an X-bearing sperm. But for the first few weeks the embryo begins developing both the male and female anatomy so that both are present at the same time. The internal ducts and the external genitalia of both sexes are present until the germ cells organise themselves into the female gonads, ie the ovaries. (For a male the same germ cells become testicles.) The formation of ovaries is quickly followed by the disintegration of the male interior ducts (spermatic cord, etc.), while the female ducts develop and thicken to become the womb, the Fallopian tubes and the top two-thirds of the vagina. The external anatomy develops to the normal female appearance, the embryonic penis ending up as the clitoris.

The surprise (and the justification for saying this route to the

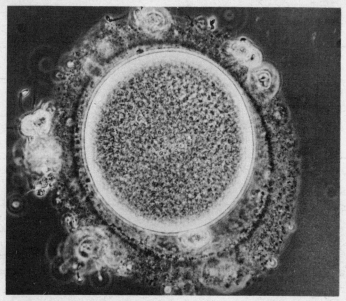

A human ovum in initial stages of fertilisation

female is the natural one) is that, even if the ovaries are removed at the earliest stages, growth still follows the femal route. If testicles are removed during the development of a male, then the development switches back to follow the female route.

To become a male means interfering with that natural route. The fight to be male begins if the sperm carries a Y chromosome. That Y forces the gonads to become testicles. The testicles are the headquarters from which the battle for a male body is fought with hormones. The testicles do not sit there passively, but first pump out a hormone which actively absorbs the female parts. That thickens the spermatic cord, and it also forces the external genitalia to develop along the male route. It causes the labia – the lips of the vulva – to fuse and create a sac into which the testicles descend.

The first step in the process whereby the Y chromosome creates testicles has recently been understood. In 1975 Stephen Wachtel of the Sloan Kettering Institute was looking for a chemical which could be the product of the Y chromosome and which would create testicles from germ cells. He searched the male embryos of frogs, birds, lemmings and humans and found one chemical common to all. A protein which for technical reasons he called H-Y antigen. It is a maleness glue. He guessed that its role was to stick to the surface of cells that would otherwise become ovaries and when they are coated with the glue they would form themselves into a testicle.

In California in 1979 Professor S. Ohno actually took the incipient ovaries from a female calf foetus and showed that H-Y antigen could convert them to testicles in a test tube.

The ovaries were dissected out of the foetus a few weeks after conception and left to grow in a solution of nutrient. One was left to grow as a control. The other had H-Y antigen added to it. That ovary came to have the structure of a testicle, the other the structure of an ovary.

Once testicles are established it is the hormones they produce which create the next steps towards maleness. After forming the testicles it seems that the Y chromosome has no other role to play.

There are many people who never complete the route to maleness and end up neither the familiar male nor female. For example, there is Mrs Daphne Went, a motherly-looking woman in her fifties. Inside her, where most women have ovaries, she has two testicles. The condition is called Testicular Feminisation Syndrome (TFS).

Her development from conception began normally enough along the male route. The egg that was to be Mrs Went was fertilised by a Y-bearing sperm. At the chromosome stage she was male, and that led to her having two normal testes. The testes secreted their first hormone and that absorbed the female parts that would otherwise become the Fallopian tubes, the womb and the top part of the vagina. Then the testes produced testosterone a powerful male hormone – but for some reason as yet unknown, her body was insensitive to it. So, apart from the womb that had been absorbed, everything developed as a female. The first sign that something had gone wrong was at puberty; she developed no pubic hair and there was no onset of menstruation.

At first she was given hormones in an attempt to bring on her periods. It wasn't until she was twenty-three that her doctor decided to send her to a gynaecologist. Mrs Went remembers how awful the interview was. 'She said, "Well, there's nothing I can do for you – nothing anybody can do for you. There's no treatment. You just haven't got a womb, and you have a very short vagina. If you intend getting married, you must explain

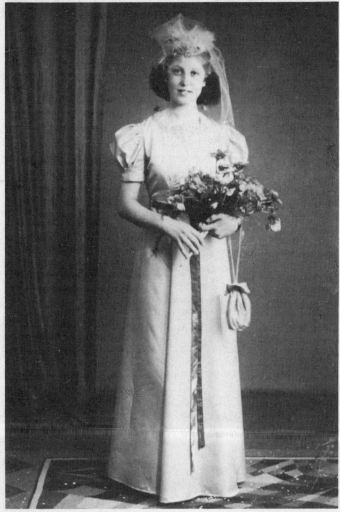

Mrs Went as a young woman

these things to your husband since there will be no children and
intercourse will be strictly limited." I found the effect for some
time after that was really hard to bear. I thought my life was over.
But you come round, and you begin to accept these things, and

when I finally met my husband he had no objection at all to adopting children, and so after we got married we adopted two. And they are now twenty-one and eighteen.'

In Mrs Went, the fight to be male was lost when her body failed to react to testosterone – nevertheless she leads an active and successful life as a woman. She is one of about 500 women in Britain who have inherited this condition.

In Cape Town, South Africa, there have been a series of remarkable people who show how complex the struggle to be male can be. 'Mr Blackwell,' a patient of Professor W. A. van Niekerk of the University of Stellenbosch, is only the 303rd patient in all of medical history to be a true hermaphrodite. He is a handsome and rather shy eighteen-year-old Bantu. Although he had a small vaginal opening as well as a penis, he was presumed a boy and brought up as a male. But when he was fourteen he developed breasts and he was sent to hospital to discover why this had happened. He was found to have an active ovary on one side of his body and an active testicle on the other. His anatomy is the result of one of his gonads becoming a testicle – which absorbed the female structure that side – while the other gonad remained an ovary – around which half a normal womb developed, because the other single testicle did not have the 'range' to absorb all the female structures.

'Mr Blackwell' had led the life of a normal boy and teenager – so he was most upset when he started to develop breasts and menstruate. That unhappiness took him to a missionary doctor who sent him to Cape Town. When he was taken into hospital he stated that he wanted to remain male – and so the female parts were removed. (He could have had the male parts removed and been made into a woman). Nevertheless he was certain he was a man, and wanted to remain one. That raises the question where the 'maleness' of his personality came from; as does a very different story from a Caribbean island.

In the south-west corner of a tropical Caribbean island live Belarminio and Benilda Batista and their family of ten children. Four of them were born as girls, grew up as girls, but, at puberty changed into muscular men. Their eldest child, Mario, now aged twenty-nine began as a girl called Antonia. Chichi, now a male nineteen-year-old, began as a girl called Isobel. Their ten-year-old, Virgilio, is in the process of changing from a female to a male. All 'changing' children were born with normal female genitalia and grew to have the normal female body shape: until, at the age of twelve, their vaginas healed over, two testicles

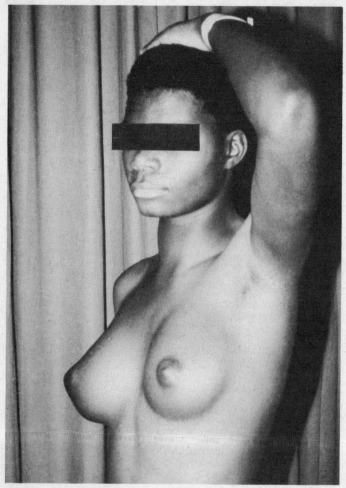

'Mr Blackwell' at time of first examination

descended and they grew full-size penises.

After their change, the boys are on average more muscular than their normal brothers. They take on the tough jobs in the local quarry. They marry and lead a normal male sexual life – even though they have not been fertile.

The Batistas are just one of twenty-three affected families in their village, in which thirty-seven children have changed. In the society of the village – a deeply religious Catholic community –

these children's change has been seen as part of God's mysterious ways. They are accepted and allowed to be themselves in a way which couldn't happen in Western society.

In conversation with Dr Gautier, director of the children's hospital on the island, the parents were quite clear about their feelings towards the children. They spoke of their pride in their new sons, of the extra money the children could bring home as boys rather than girls; and they insisted that the children's adjustment to their new gender-roles was immediate. Benilda admitted having had feelings of sadness and worry; but, supported by a devout community, she came to see the phenomenon as God's will: 'If *we* made children with our own hands we would make them perfect, beautiful and complete. But God knows what he's doing.'

Although girls had been changing into boys since 1930, it was not known outside the district until the first doctor went on holiday there. He published his findings about the children, in an obscure Spanish journal, where it lay unnoticed until 1972. Dr Gautier's attention was originally drawn by a patient who had been in his hospital when about eight years old, and whose behaviour had then seemed completely female. And some time later he met that person working in the mountains cutting wood, and his behaviour was as a male. Dr Gautier was so surprised that he and a group of scientists started to investigate the change and how it came about.

When the scientists put all the family pedigrees together, they began to see the interrelationship between one family and the next. They ended up with an enormous family tree, showing twenty-three families going back seven generations to one woman – Altagracia Carrasco. She lived in the mid-nineteenth century, and she is the common ancestor of all the affected families. The mutant gene has been passed down from her – but only shows when both parents carry it. How these children develop in the womb has been worked out by the scientists, and it gives a new twist to the story of how male genitalia form.

The egg is fertilised by a Y sperm, and it first develops to a foetus with normal testes. Perfectly normally, they absorb the female parts, and testosterone preserves the male ducts. But in these children's cases, it doesn't change the external anatomy, because, in their bodies the children miss a critical chemical step.

Normal men are able to process cholesterol through to testosterone – and on to a mysterious hormone called dihydro-

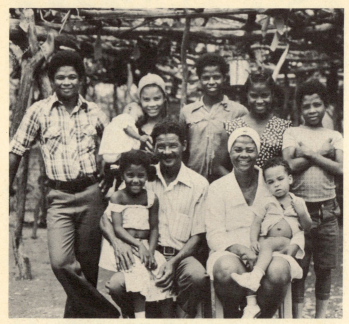

The Batista family: Mario (extreme left) *and Chichi* (centre of back row) *both began life as girls – as Antonia and Isobel respectively.*

testosterone. No one knew what its function was. But because the Caribbean children cannot make it, and because injecting it into them stimulates their genital growth, it is clear now that dihydrotestosterone creates the male external anatomy. The pubertal surge of testosterone in these children forces up the dihydrotestosterone level and growth that should have happened ten years before, in the mother's womb, takes place at last.

The important point that emerges from this work is that the children's brains were exposed to a normal male level of testosterone before and after birth. That suggests very strongly that their readiness to adopt male roles is explained by testosterone programming masculinity into their brains. This explanation flew in the face of most scientific belief, because it suggested that female brains and male brains are different at birth. It is a controversial area of study. Are boys born already programmed to find girls erotically stimulating, or do they learn it? Are girls born with a maternal instinct – or do they learn it? Most scientists would say these differences in sex role and behaviour are learnt.

There is no doubt we do behave differently to baby boys than to baby girls and thereby we may teach the children to be different. At Sussex University, Caroline Smith has been studying how women play with a young child (aged about six months) that they haven't met before. The subtlety of the experiment is that the children are often not the sex they appear to be. A boy baby may often be dressed as a little girl. That's so she could rule out the possibility that the baby itself was calling forth reactions from the woman.

She found that the toys offered to the babies were influenced by the child's presumed sex. Typically a boy was handed a plastic squeezy hammer and a girl a doll. The women encouraged boys to be active and stimulated them by jiggling them around. They talked more to children they presumed to be girls, tried to calm them and told them how pretty they were. It seems we do try to teach our children to be different.

That the sex role is learnt was a theory that was first put forward by John Money at Johns Hopkins University hospital in Baltimore. The theory has been accepted for the last twenty years. Dr Money said that not only did a child learn its sex, but that once learnt it could not change it. He was treating children who had been assigned the wrong sex at birth. He tried to help them change into their correct sex, the one they could be fertile in. He found they could not accept a change but would have a nervous breakdown.

Money came to believe that, between birth and the age of two, the child could learn to be either sex, but after two it became 'fixed' in its sexual identity. It seemed to him and his co-worker, Anke Ehrhardt, that children were born equally able to learn to be a boy or a girl.

One of his most important cases, the one which has been most influential on the medical profession's thinking, was the loss of a penis by a baby male, one of a pair of male twins. The second child accidentally lost most of his penis at his circumcision. After much anguish about what to do the parents came to Money, who advised them to have the child castrated and to bring it up as a girl. Breasts and an artificial vagina would be created by hormones and surgery as the need arose. That was the course the parents took, and Money claimed that the child learnt very successfully to be a girl. Recently, the success of this particular case has been disputed. At the age of sixteen the child feels suicidal, is under psychiatric care, and does not like wearing girl's clothes. Nevertheless it's still generally held that Money's idea was correct; and it is part of medical practice today that if a male is born with a very small penis (called a micropenis) then the child will have a better life if converted to a 'girl'.

To a consultant who takes such decisions at a London children's hospital, it is a tragic situation, one of trying to make the best of a bad job: 'One has to balance life as a male, without a penis, versus life as a female, who has no uterus and no possibility of fertility, and who at the time of adolescence will need oestrogen therapy to produce breast development. Obviously this is a difficult decision. I think most parents would feel that, in the new-born period, where there hasn't been any definite decision on the gender, life for their child would be better as a girl rather than as a boy.' That micropenis boys usually grow up to be happy females is powerful evidence that we do learn our sex, that there is no significant difference between the male and female brain at birth.

But in the early seventies at the University of California in Los Angeles, experimental work began that casts doubt on the idea that sexual behaviour is all learning. Professor Roger Gorski has been studying what controls the way rats copulate. The normal response of the female rat to being mounted is to arch her back. If a male is mounted by a bigger more dominant rat he doesn't arch. Gorski has found he can give female sexual behaviour to an otherwise seemingly normal male rat. He deprives a male rat of testosterone during a critical period just *after* birth. The rats so treated grow normally and at first there is no way the effect of that deprivation could be detected. But those males grow up to behave as females. They have no male libido, and behave sexually exactly as females would, including arching the back when mounted.

To find what the cause of the differences in behaviour could be, Gorski's team have been sectioning rat brains, staining them and searching for a difference between rats with male behaviour and those with female behaviour. They searched for years unsuccessfully. Now they have found a difference. In a slice across a male rat brain about half-way back, there is a tiny centre that stains blue. In a female brain that centre is smaller. It is the same in a 'feminised' male. In rats, at least, the female brain is different from the male one.

A mechanism by which brain difference arises has been recently discovered by Dr Toran Allerand at Columbia University, New York. She dissects out that 'sex centre' from the brain of a foetal mouse and keeps the tiny fragment of brain alive in drops of liquid. Half of the brain fragment is grown in fluids to which testosterone has been added.

After eight days, the half that is growing in the testosterone has developed a thick network of nerve fibres richly inter-connected. The half grown in the female environment, without testosterone, is different. There are only half the number of cells, and there is less connection. This lack of development is not true for other areas of the brain, such as those which might contain memory and intelligence. It is only true for the tiny centre that is thought to control sex behaviour. One speculation is that testosterone prevents cell death and so preserves the male sex centre. However that may be, the fact is that testosterone leads to a large centre and lack of it to a small one.

Could this also apply to humans? Dr Gorski's reply is cautious. 'This is a difficult question to answer. Of course, it's a focus of a great deal of research. But, certainly, the concept that we can change the sex of the brain is not restricted only to the rat. It has been demonstrated in other animals, in other rodents, and in addition, to the rhesus monkey, and other types of monkeys. And there is some suggestion from the clinical litera-ture that this may in fact apply to the human being.'

The most important parts of that clinical literature are the work of Professor Gerd Dörner. He believes the 'female' be-haviour of the feminised male is part of the explanation of human male homosexuality. He works in East Berlin at the Institute for Experimental Hormone Research at Humboldt University. In 1968, with a big research team, he began looking for a sex centre which, if malformed, he believed could result in homosexuality. He began by looking for the sex centre in rats, and he had found it before Gorski. When he destroyed a small particular part of the brain of a newborn male rat, he could make the male behave as a female. In his terms, it became homosexual.

What Professor Dörner is now doing is trying to show that humans do have a sex centre – and that male homosexuals have a female one. He has developed a test in which the brain of a male homosexual is fooled into thinking it is in a woman's body. The theory is that an injection of oestrogen into the homosexual's body looks to the brain like the signal from a womb after ovulation. The signals that his brain sends back down to this 'phantom' womb reveals the sex of the brain. Samples of blood are taken during the next four days, and the amount of female ovulation-inducing hormone – called LH – is measured. In tests with twenty homosexuals Dörner found their brains responded to the oestrogen as a woman's would – with an LH surge. Non-homosexual males subjected to the same treatment had no such reaction to phantom wombs. This work has not been substantiated by being repeated in other laboratories, and many scientists do not accept it.

As another way of proving his views. Dörner is now studying mothers in their fourth month of pregnancy, the time which he believes is the critical period for the formation of a male sex centre. For various medical reasons, some pregnant women have samples of fluid taken from the womb. Dörner gets samples from such women, and uses them to measure the testosterone level in their wombs. Should it be low, he plans to watch the future behaviour of that child (if it is male). In the process he expects to prove that a low testosterone in the womb leads to male homosexuality. If he does get that proof he thinks the next step might be to inject more testosterone – and so prevent homosexuality, at least in part. He sees it as a simple matter of 'correcting' abnormalities in sex hormone levels. The moral implications, he insists, are for society in general to decide.

This highly controversial approach to homosexuality fits particularly well with the East German view that there is a definable male, and that deviation from that definition should be corrected. Science and politics are more interwoven in the communist bloc than elswhere. Dörner has been given major awards by East German academics, who welcome his findings. Although the tone and implication of his work are unwelcome to the West, his ideas are being seriously, if reluctantly, considered here.

Meanwhile he is taking his experiments along a new direction. For two separate hour-long periods each day, pregnant rats are subjected to the stress of being unable to move while exposed to fierce arc-lamps. Stress causes the production of adrenalin, and one of the effects of adrenalin is to suppress the action of the testicles. Dörner's idea is that male foetuses in the rats under stress will be more likely to grow up to be homosexual. He says that, after many experiments, he can clearly show that there is a decrease in the testosterone level of such foetuses. And there is a possibility that the same mechanism works in humans.

He has looked at the frequencies of male homosexuals born during the especially stressful situation in Germany during the Second World War, and has compared them with those that were born six years before and six years afterwards. In a sample of about 500 cases he claims to have found that about twice as many male homosexuals were born during the war as compared to during the six years immediately before or afterwards. This may be an indication, he cautiously says, that stress can be an important factor in bringing about permanent changes of sex hormones, and may induce permanent changes in the offspring.

Not everybody is happy with this evidence. Dr Anke Ehrhardt, for example, who worked with John Money on the twins, feels that Dörner has made the jump from rat behaviour to human homosexuality in an unacceptable way. She points out that there was a time when a researcher found higher levels of testosterone in heterosexual males than in controls. 'It took about fifteen years for other investigators to refute that finding. It probably had something to do with the sample selection. So the finding which Dörner claims just has to be established by other investigators.'

Professor Roger Gorski also wants to wait and see: 'The work that Dörner is doing could give us a solid answer as to whether or not there is dependence on hormones in homosexual behaviour, but I think the verdict is not in yet.'

Mrs Went and 'Mr Blackwell's' feelings are very relevant to this question, and to the whole problem of whether the male and female roles are inherent or learnt. 'Mr Blackwell' used to ovulate and menstruate before his operation. His whole hormonal profile was completely female – and that would imply that he would have a 'female' sex centre in his brain – if such a centre exists in humans. Yet in spite of a female brain Mr Blackwell is psychosexually a very ordinary boy with male attitudes to girl-friends. His condition does not give support to the idea that a feminised brain controls his behaviour.

Nor do Mrs Went's feelings agree with the concept of an inherent male or female brain. During her development and through her life her testicles have surrounded her brain with normal male levels of testosterone. So her brain should be male. That was tested by giving her the 'phantom womb' tests: her brain responded in the characteristic male way. So if behaviour is inherent she could be expected to have male feelings. But by her own testimony she never at any time felt masculine in any way. Her femininity was plainly learnt.

However, the behaviour of the Caribbean children paradoxically supports the idea that sexual behaviour is inborn. All the children had had usual levels of testosterone while developing in the womb. The thirty-seven 'girls' spontaneously felt a desire to be male. That seems to show that hormones do pre-programme the male brain with masculine behaviour before birth. Did this, as it appears, override the sex they had been taught? Or was their upbringing special? Was their upbringing preparing them for the change because their parents had learnt to recognise their condition from the slightly enlarged clitoris, a symptom which had become well-known in the village?

It is not easy to take a view about this now as, since 1977, all the children have been identified and are being brought up as boys – and parents who carry the gene are being given genetic counselling so it will not happen again. But the parents of the Batista family are quite certain they treated their children who changed exactly like other girls when they were young. It is possible that what happened in the village would not apply to other cultures. There, the families were able to accept the children's change without crushing feelings of guilt and shame.

What of the scientists working with these families? Do they think that it is generally true that these male hormones known as androgens play a major role in pre-programming human sexual behaviour? The Director of the team, Dr Imperato-McGinley, thinks the question remains unanswered, certainly as far as humans are concerned.

'It has been thought that in man, unlike the animals, our hormones play a very small role. When we came across these patients we were rather shocked, because they appeared to disprove the dictum of twenty years. Now, that is not to say that the sex of rearing is not important. We don't mean to say it at all. What we mean to say is that we now have to recognise that, before birth, hormones *do* play a role in gender-identity formation.'

So where does masculinity and femininity come from? Must we compromise by saying that adult sexuality is the result of pre-birth programming, and the interaction of that partly formed gender-identity with the way we are brought up? It is not possible at this stage to give a better answer. How we grow to be male and female physically in the womb is now a relatively objective science. But human behaviour is so complex and so individual that trying to unravel any threads of understanding of male and female behaviour after birth becomes progressively misty. It now seems likely that men and women are born with differences in their brains. We don't know much about what effect that has or if those differences are important. The real understanding has yet to come.

The differences in human behaviour stem from the activities of the brain. Not only are there differences between sexes and between individuals, but the amounts of chemicals producing those different behaviour patterns in any one individual are constantly changing. Those chemicals, and their interactions, are programmed by genes, genetic information that makes up the DNA that sits in the nucleus of every cell. The central core of medical research, cell biology, begins to emerge.

But that's not all. Each bundle of cells, calling itself a human, reacts with an alien environment. It must defend itself against other bundles of cells, sometimes also calling themselves humans but also sometimes quite different bundles – known as, say, lions and tigers, sharks and crocodiles, or mosquitoes and fleas, or bacteria, or viruses. In fact, a bacterium is only a single cell and a virus is merely a package of DNA with hardly any other cell material around it. Nonetheless each organism, large or small, does battle with all the other organisms according to its own genetic code. It does this in a physical environment in which changes in temperature and pressure and the presence or absence of certain gases, are all-important to it.

It was in these circumstances that one of the classic detective stories unfolded. There was death, inexplicable clues, a little bit of luck, great skill and much systematic slogging on the part of an international team of investigators. To begin with, one of the protagonists was unknown. It took an extraordinary event for it to appear.

7 The Hunt for the Legion Killer

Dominic Flessati

In 1976 the United States of America were celebrating their Bicentennial – the 200th anniversary of the Declaration of Independence. At the centre of nationwide celebrations was Philadelphia, the city where the Declaration had been drawn up and where the new Republic's first Congress had met. Many distinguished visitors were expected to visit 'Freedom City' that year, among them the President of the United States, Gerald Ford, the President of France, and the Queen of England. Ordinary tourists and sight-seers were expected in millions, and a summer-long season of entertainments had been planned for them.

On 21 July an extrovert and colourful group of visitors arrived in Philadelphia. They wore uniform blue blazers and jaunty forage caps that proclaimed them to be members of the Pennsylvania Department of the American Legion, the national association of military veterans. They were holding their annual convention 2500 strong. The convention centre was the Bellevue-Stratford, the city's most venerable and famous hotel. Many of the Legion delegates and their wives stayed in the hotel, where the formal sessions were also held – to hear keynote speeches and annual reports, to make presentations and elect officers. There were also a grand ball and plenty of parties in which to enjoy the hospitality and good cheer typical of the Legion.

On Saturday 24 July the Legionnaires departed for their homes in hundreds of towns and villages across the large and populous state of Pennsylvania. A few were feeling ill – not just the expected hangovers and indigestions – but something worse and rather strange. More fell ill after getting home. In the town of Bloomsburg, three Legionnaires were taken to hospital with fever. It was diagnosed as typhoid; but within hours one of them, William Baird, died of 'acute lung failure'.

On Friday 30 July the Bloomsburg physician, Dr Ernest

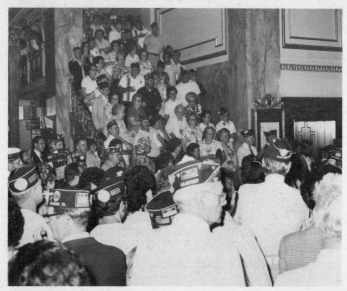

The lobby of the Belevue-Stratford Hotel, Philadelphia, July 1976. Of the American Legion delegates and their wives many were to fall mysteriously ill and 31 were to die.

Campbell, realising that all three patients had been to a convention in Philadelphia, called the State Health Department to report the matter but was told they were shut until Monday. Over that weekend the American Legion's State Adjutant, Ed Hoak, was visiting Legion posts in the Pittsburgh area. He heard of a number of comrades being ill, and of the sudden death of one whom he had seen just the week before at the Convention. On Sunday evening he went to his office in the Legion's State HQ and telephoned Legion officers in other parts of the state: everywhere the picture was the same: dozens of Legionnaires were ill, as were some of their wives; at least five more had died. Some victims were elderly but others were vigorous men in their forties.

At 8.30 on Monday morning Hoak got through to Dr William Shrack, at the Health Department in Harrisburg, the State capital, and reported his findings. At last the alarm was sounded: a statewide health alert was issued. Hoak, anxious to warn his Legionnaires to seek medical help the moment they felt ill, called a press conference. By then he knew of twelve deaths. Then

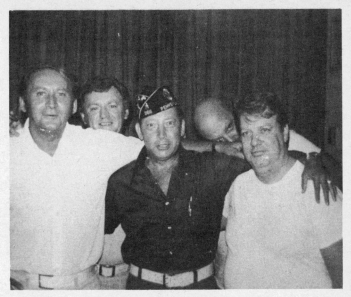

Old comrades at the Philadelphia Convention: a few days later John B. Ralph (second from left) *and James T. Dolan* (right) *were dead.*

phone calls started to pour in, from all over the State, with news of more cases. An operations room was set up which worked until the early hours of the morning, listing the names and addresses of sick Legionnaires, the hospitals to which they had been taken – or the morgues.

Meanwhile, on that same morning of 2 August the State Health authorities decided they could not handle the emergency alone. They sent a call for help to the Center for Disease Control in Atlanta, Georgia. CDC, as it is known, is a Federal agency for fighting infectious disease. It is the largest in the world. It employs 3500 doctors and scientists. At its Atlanta HQ a complex of buildings contains dozens of specialised labs doing research into the deadliest micro-organisms known to mankind – age-old scourges like leprosy, small-pox and rabies, as well as more recently-discovered ones like Lassa fever. To prevent any infection spreading, each lab is segregated from the others and restricted to the people who work in it. A special pass is needed to open its door. Once inside researchers spend their lives working under artificial light, and breathing filtered air, and no windows or doors give direct access to the outside world.

One of CDC's facilities is a corps of eighty Epidemic Intelligence Officers. These are young doctors who wish to pursue a career in public health. While on a two-year training course at CDC they are also on stand-by to investigate epidemics anywhere in the country. In response to the call for help from Pennsylvania on 2 August three EIS officers were despatched at once. In the evening the Director of CDC, Dr David Sencer, called a meeting to review the situation, and decided that because of the growing size of the problem a staff epidemiologist should be sent to take charge. The man chosen was Dr David Fraser. It was to turn into the most intensive investigation ever mounted by CDC.

By 3 August when Fraser set up his HQ in Harrisburg, the death toll had reached sixteen. As he began to hand out tasks he realised that he would need yet more help. The State health staff were already fully deployed. Reinforcements were sent from CDC until he had a total of thirty-one EIS officers at work. Their first task was to characterise the disease which so far had displayed baffling and contradictory symptoms; then to find out who had got it, when they had got it – and where. They fanned out over Pennsylvania, visiting 300 hospitals, to track down every single case and interview survivors about symptoms.

For many victims, such as Thomas Payne, the onset had not been very dramatic; he just felt unusually tired, then as it progressed, achey, as if he was getting the flu. But soon he developed pain in the stomach and groin, and was running a fever of 104°F. Then he began to have trouble breathing. He was given oxygen. A range of clinical tests failed to yield a clue as to the cause. Without a diagnosis, his doctors began to give him massive doses of penicillin – the last thing he remembers clearly; his fever was still going up – it was constantly checked on a rectal thermometer. Afterwards they told him that it had peaked at 107.4 degrees. He had to be sponged down with cold water to try and control the fever.

Jim Kelly's experience had been somewhat milder, but still had significant features: he had only been at the Convention in Philadelphia for one day – the Friday! He began to feel ill on the Saturday with a bad headache and pains in the stomach. By Sunday his chest was hurting – just as if he had a heavy cold – and his kidneys were so sore he could hardly bear to lie on his back: 'There were several times while I was in bed that I was so damned sore that I wished I could die.'

From dozens of interviews Dr Fraser and his team at last

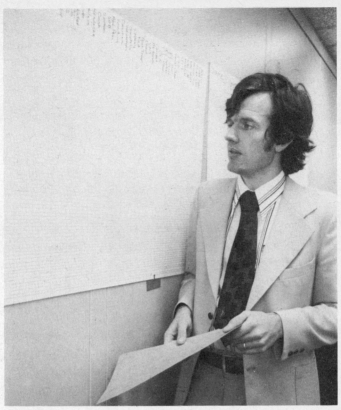

Dr David Fraser, the young investigator from the Center for Disease Control in Atlanta, checking the list of victims and their symptoms.

acquired a reliable picture of the disease. It was primarily a pneumonia, that is an inflammation of the lungs, but kidneys and liver were also commonly involved. At the beginning, the illness was characterised by a low-grade fever, headaches, and muscle aches. Then the fever rose rapidly, often to 104 or 105 degrees, and in many cases was associated with shaking chills. Many patients had a cough but it was often dry. Many had diarrhoea – many more than one would expect with pneumonia. Some patients were exceptionally confused – more confused than would be expected with their degree of fever. The disease went on for seven to ten days, and about one in six patients died.

As to where they had got the disease, the Bellevue-Stratford

Hotel, the Convention HQ, was heavily implicated. Legion-naires who got sick were more likely to have stayed there than at other hotels; and those who had stayed at other hotels were more likely to get sick the longer they spent in the Bellevue-Stratford at meetings and parties. It also turned out that many of the sick were not Legionnaires or their wives at all: seventy-two of them had been in the Bellevue-Stratford for other reasons or were merely passers-by on Broad Street in front of the hotel.

During the Convention the Legion had staged a parade which passed along Broad Street. One woman went in to watch it from a second-floor window of the Bellevue-Stratford. She was only there three hours but she got sick and died. She was especially unlucky because analysis of the interview data showed that women were far less likely to get it than men. Another risk factor was age – older Legionnaires were likelier to get ill than younger ones; and smokers were at higher risk than non-smokers.

But what was the cause of the disease? Routine tests in local hospitals had found none of the commoner bacteria or viruses that would account for the symptoms. So clinical samples were collected and rushed by police cars and helicopters to the Pennsylvania State labs and to those at CDC in Atlanta. By 4 August there were twenty-one dead, so the samples were handled with great care, inside safety cabinets under sterilising ultra-violet light.

Lung tissue from dead Legionnaires, divided into tiny portions, was distributed among a number of CDC labs, and tested for the presence of micro-organisms. Each lab used its own special procedures. In the pathology lab they embedded slivers of lung in wax and sliced them up with a microtome into almost transparent, thin sections. On a glass slide and suitably stained they might reveal the presence of one of the dozen different bacteria, viruses, or fungi known to cause pneumonia. The pathologists used a whole range of different dyes to prepare hundreds of slides and examined them with meticulous care. They saw plenty of dark-stained inflammatory cells inside the lung tissue – the body's reaction to attack – but of a micro-organism causing the reaction they saw no trace.

In other labs bacteriologists were spreading lung material from dead Legionnaires onto culture plates to see if colonies of bacteria would grow on them – bacteria which might then be identified as disease-causing organisms. They did over 400 individual tests using fourteen different kinds of nutrient culture medium, but no disease-causing bacteria grew up on the plates.

Meanwhile in the virology labs even trickier procedures were being followed. Most viruses will not grow on artificial culture media. Lung or other material had to be inoculated into eggs with live embryos or into living guinea-pigs and mice. Again they did over 400 tests, each lasting several days. It was all negative – no virus was isolated.

The search was widened to less likely areas. Dr Joseph McDade was in charge of a lab that works on micro-organisms called rickettsias. These are smaller than bacteria but larger than viruses. One rickettsia, *Coxiella burnetii,* causes a disease called Q-fever, a form of pneumonia. It was not really like the disease seen in Philadelphia but McDade was asked to test for it.

Rickettsias, like viruses, will only grow in living hosts. To isolate them requires a painstaking and time-consuming procedure. Guinea-pigs were inoculated with lung tissue from Philadelphia victims, and then were kept under observation for a few days. Some developed a fever, and were killed and autopsied. Organs such as the spleen were removed. If any rickettsias were present they would be concentrated in the spleen. This was ground up with pestle and mortar and made into a fluid suspension. A tiny amount of the suspension was inoculated into eggs containing live chick embryos. By incubating the eggs for up to ten days, any rickettsias present were given a chance to multiply inside the yolk-sacs, and so be easier to isolate and identify.

Yolk-sacs of embryos that had died after the third day were taken out and smeared on slides. Dr McDade examined them under a microscope, along with other slides smeared with spleen tissue from the guinea-pigs. They had all been stained with a dye which should make rickettsias visible, but McDade found none. All he saw was an occasional rod-shaped organism, probably a bacterium – a contaminant of no significance in his search for rickettsias. He reported that whatever had killed the Legionnaires it was not the Q-fever rickettsia.

While all this work was going on the death toll had risen to twenty-four. But on 6 August there had been some good news to announce at the daily press conference held by the investigating team in Harrisburg: there were no new cases to report. The disease was not spreading person to person among the Legionnaires' families. This meant that whatever the cause, all the victims had been exposed to it in the same place and roughly at the same time – the days of the Convention in Philadelphia. It was a single-source outbreak.

This, together with the failure of the micro-biologists to find anything, strengthened a suspicion that the cause might be a toxic substance – a poison of some sort. CDC toxicologists took up the hunt. If a toxic substance was the killer then the field to be searched was very wide. There are about thirty metallic elements which can be toxic, and about 35,000 organic compounds. Most of these could be screened out by general testing, but a special search was made for substances known to produce symptoms like those seen in Philadelphia.

Among the metals, nickel was a prime suspect. To test for it they used the technique of atomic absorption spectrophotometry on batches of blood samples from Legionnaires. They found nothing. On another type of test they did find abnormal amounts of nickel in lung samples – only to discover that it came from the scalpels used to cut them up. When plastic knives were substituted for the scalpels, the test turned out negative.

When it came to testing for toxic organic substances CDC again tried to narrow down the field to a few of the likelier suspects, by searching the computerised files at the National Library of Medicine in Washington which holds toxicity data on 35,000 organic compounds. A likely suspect was paraquat, a deadly weedkiller. It was thought that paraquat could have been used around trees outside the Bellevue-Stratford Hotel. Liquid chromatography was used to search for paraquat in urine samples from sick Legionnaires. The technique could detect the tiniest traces of the poison – but none was found.

There was nothing for it but to screen samples by wide-spectrum methods looking for traces of something significant. The toxicologists had got their share of lung tissue from dead Legionnaires. They too crushed up tiny portions and put them into suspension. Gas chromatography was used to detect unusual compounds in the lung. The GC apparatus produces a chart on which the various organic substances in a sample appear as peaks of different height on a continuously traced line. By comparing the trace of a Legion victim with that from a normal control lung some significant difference might be found. If an unusual compound did show up it was put into a mass spectrometer to get an even more detailed analysis of its composition. The result was put into a computer to be compared with profiles of over 30,000 compounds on file. One sample aroused great excitement when found to contain a heavily chlorinated compound but it turned out to belong to a woman who had worked for years in a dry cleaning firm.

Day after day – and often long into the night – the toxicologists worked, poring over the charts, some of which were so long they had to be laid out on laboratory floors. Meanwhile, in Philadelphia itself the field team were checking the Bellevue-Stratford and its neighbourhood for clues to an environmental poison. They also checked other bars and restaurants frequented by the Legionnaires during the Convention. Over a thousand samples were collected and sent to CDC for analysis: samples of water from bedrooms, kitchens, and cooling systems, or that had once been ice for drinks; of dust from various rooms, from carpets and lift-shafts; insect debris from ventilation grilles; pigeon droppings; household disinfectants and cleaning fluids; pesticides and insecticides; plastics and resins which might have given off fumes when heated. Even the souvenir pack distributed to the Legionnaires – containing literature, badges and cigarettes – came under suspicion. But after months of work, at a cost of 90,000 man-hours and two-million dollars, the world's top disease detectives had failed to account for the 221 cases of severe disease and thirty-four deaths.

Dr Fraser and his field team retreated back to Atlanta, weary and baffled. The press proclaimed their failure in merciless headlines. There were even accusations of a cover-up for incompetence. A Congressional committee, chaired by Representative John M. Murphy, investigated the actions of Dr Fraser and his colleagues. Murphy suggested that an anti-military madman had murdered the nation's veterans. The press were spurred to wilder excesses. An identikit picture of a man seen hanging around the Convention – presumably the murderer – was published. The FBI and the CIA were urged to investigate. . . .

More soberly, in mid-December 1976, CDC compiled a report summarising its investigations so far. It listed the thousands of negative tests, and in particular spelled out the failure of the toxicologists on whom the main hope had been pinned. Among those who read the report was Dr Joseph McDade of the rickettsia lab. It stirred a nagging doubt. He had never been able to show what had caused the fever in the guinea-pigs he had inoculated with material from dead Legionnaires. There was a remote possibility that the rod-shaped organisms he had seen on his slides had in fact been the cause of the fever in the animals and therefore of the Legionnaires' disease.

Two days after Christmas 1976, McDade came to his lab and in the holiday quiet started looking again at the slides prepared four months earlier with smears of yolk-sac and guinea-pig spleen. Back in August he had only seen the occasional rod-shaped organism, stained red. Now, manipulating the knob on his microscope to change his field of view, after fifteen minutes on the very first slide he happened upon a whole cluster of the rods. This was a startling find. In such numbers these organisms could well have caused the guinea-pigs' illness – and the Legionnaires'. But had they?

The way to find out was to see if blood serum from sick Legionnaires contained antibody to these rod-shaped organisms. He used a test known as the Indirect Fluorescent Antibody test – IFA for short – in which you use glass slides with a row of shallow wells. In each well you put a speck of fresh yolk-sac containing invading organisms – in McDade's test, the rods. A drop of blood serum from one of the patients is added. If there is antibody to the rods in the blood it will bind to them – it is the function of antibody to immobilise invading organisms. Then a fluorescent dye is added. If antibody is present the dye will stain it. The slides are then examined with a microscope under ultraviolet light. Under this the dye fluoresces, revealing the antibody locked to the rods as bright green blobs against a dark background. This is just what McDade saw when he did the IFA test with Legionnaires' blood. At last he had found the Legion killer!

McDade's reaction, recalled later, seems modest: 'Those findings came over several weeks, so there was never really one given day when we thought for certain that we had found the cause of the disease. I just remember it as being a very exciting time, a very fast-moving time, and a very uncertain time. I distinctly remember feeling I hope I'm right.'

He *was* right. He had found the killer – but what exactly was it? In shape and size it looked like a bacterium, but it had failed to grow on nutrient media on which bacteria normally thrive and so reveal themselves. Another CDC bacteriologist, Dr Robert Weaver, set out to try and grow it on a range of different media, including the ones used back in August 1976. He tried seventeen without success. Finally he tried one that had been suggested by colleages in a neighbouring lab, who used it to grow the bacteria that cause gonorrhoea. He put a drop of yolk-sac suspension in the middle of the plate and left it there instead of spreading it out in the usual way over the whole surface. He hoped that by leaving the suspension concentrated the organisms would have a better chance of multiplying. After a few days' incubation a white

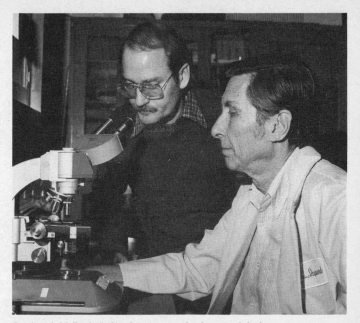

Dr Joseph McDade (left), *the scientist who discovered the bacterium causing Legionnaires' disease, with Dr Charles Shepard, head of the rickettsia laboratory in which he worked at CDC Atlanta.*

colony of the rods appeared. It was about the size of a penny, and was unmistakable. This proved the killer organism was a bacterium. But why was it so hard to grow?

This problem was studied by two more CDC men, Dr John Feeley and Dr George Gorman. They analysed the medium Weaver had used – it is called Muller-Hinton agar – and found it was made of three ingredients: agar, blood haemoglobin, and a proprietary mixture called IsoVitalex. In a series of experiments they discovered that it was the iron contained in the haemoglobin that McDade's bacterium needed; and in the IsoVitalex, which contained eleven ingredients, only one, an amino-acid called cysteine, was essential for the bacterium's growth. It was a very fastidious feeder indeed.

For the Muller-Hinton agar Feeley and Gorman substituted another containing a good helping of the two essential ingredients – iron and cysteine. On this McDade's bacterium flourished even better.

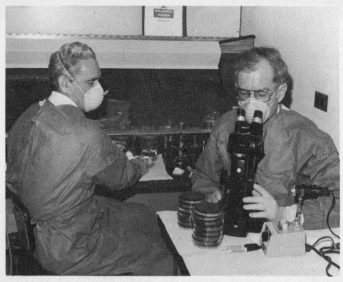

Dr George Gorman and Dr John Feeley examining culture plates to see if they have begun to grow the bacterium causing Legionnaries' disease. Early failure to do so held up the investigation for months.

Meanwhile Dr Francis Chandler and his colleagues in the pathology lab were investigating why it had been so difficult to see the bacterium in lung tissue stained with the usual dyes for bacteria – after all they had tried enough of them. They tried again, using less conventional techniques. One had been developed more than fifty years before to stain the spirochaetes that cause syphilis. It was a yellow stain – and it worked! McDade's bacteria showed up under the microscope as brown rods – much easier to spot.

Given the bacterium's unusual characteristics, a suspicion began to grow: were they dealing with a previously unknown species? The answer came from Dr Don Brenner's lab at CDC. A bacterium is a single-cell organism, and inside each one there is a chromosome in the form of a double strand of DNA – the genetic material. The DNA can be extracted from the bacterial cells and put into solution. Under certain conditions, if this solution is heated the double strands split apart into single strands. If the solution is cooled down, and then incubated, the single strands reassociate into double ones. If DNA from one

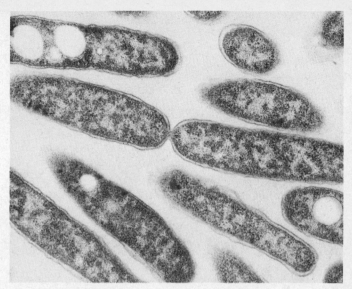

The cause of Legionnaires' disease: the rod-shaped bacterium Legionella pneumophila *magnified 40,000 times under an electron microscope.*

species of bacterium is mixed with DNA from another, and then heated, all the strands will split apart. When cooled, some strands from one species will reassociate with strands from the other to form double hybrid strands. The closer the two species are related, the greater the proportion of hybrid strands that form. If more than seventy per cent hybridise, then the two species are the same.

Dr Brenner's lab used this DNA hybridisation technique to see whether McDade's bacterium was related to any previously known species – or whether it was indeed new. They tried to get McDade's bacterium to hybridise with a wide range of known bacteria. In none of the tests did any significant hybridisation take place. This confirmed that McDade's bacterium constituted a new species, indeed a new genus. They called the genus *Legionella,* and the species *pneumophila.*

The killer's identity was now fully established but the epidemiologists still needed to solve two major problems: how did *Legionella* infect its victims? And where was it coming from? Epidemics can be spread in a limited number of ways, including person to person, through insect bites, or through contaminated food or water. There was no evidence for any of these in Philadelphia, apart from some slight evidence involving water. There was evidence, however, that the disease might have been spread through the air. People who spent more time in the lobby of the Bellevue-Stratford Hotel were more likely to get sick than those who spent less time there. And the more time people had spent on the pavement in front of the hotel, the likelier they were to get sick – the pavement was only a few feet away from the lobby. It seemed possible that the agent had somehow contaminated the air in the lobby and that people who breathed it in became ill. The Bellevue-Stratford Hotel had an air-conditioning system but, though it was thoroughly examined, nothing could be found to prove it had spread the infection. Yet a clue that air-conditioning could be a mode of spread came from an unexpected quarter.

Over the years CDC has an impressive record of success in identifying the cause of epidemics, but it has also sometimes failed. One such failure occurred in 1968, at Pontiac, a town in Michigan. There was an outbreak of disease in the County Health Department, a two-storey brick building which housed various facilities, including child health and dental clinics. About 100 people worked there as receptionists, nurses, and doctors. In 1968 there was a heat-wave at the end of June, and the outbreak exploded on 2 July. One of the women in the typing pool, Marylee Doyle, developed typical symptoms: 'I started getting a headache and I thought maybe I was going to have a migraine. And then I began to ache all over, and pretty soon my lunch wasn't setting too well, and my skin started feeling funny, and I thought this is a terrible time of the year to come down with the flu'.

Marylee's flu-like symptoms were shared by ninety-four other employees and by forty-nine visitors to the clinics. The building was emptied on 4 July, and two EIS officers from CDC arrived: 'One of the investigators,' recalls Marylee, 'was a young man who came and looked at the case reports, talked to some of us, and decided that it was more or less a case of mass hysteria. I think it was maybe three days later he was taken out of Oakland County by ambulance to the plane and shipped back to Atlanta. He kind of caught our mass hysteria.'

The CDC man, together with his colleague, had worked in the building over the weekend when the air conditioning was off. On Monday it was switched on, and they fell ill on Tuesday. When a new team arrived from Atlanta they put cages of guinea-

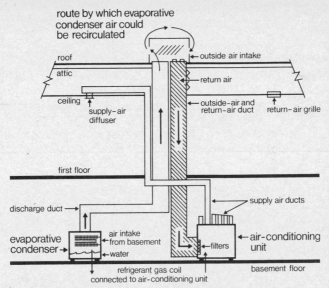

route by which evaporative
condenser air could
be recirculated

*The air conditioning system of the County Health Department, Pontiac,
Michigan: this was the first place where scientists got evidence that* Legionella
pneumophila *can infect humans through such systems.*

pigs around the Health Department building. The animals
developed fever within two or three days. At post-mortem their
lungs were found covered with blister-like nodules. But extensive lab tests failed to find a causative micro-organism – just
as they failed to find anything in swabs and specimens taken
from the human patients. Fortunately the Pontiac fever in
humans was as brief as it was sudden: within two or three days
most were on the way to rcovery, and no one died.

It did look as though they had been infected through the air.
The layout of the air-conditioning plant in the building turned
out to be significant. One unit pumps cool air into the offices
through a series of ducts. The air is cooled by passing it over
coils full of refrigerant gas. As it cools the air, the gas itself gets
hot, and so it is passed into an adjoining unit called an evaporative condenser. Here the hot gas circulates through a coil onto
which cold water is sprayed. On the hot coil the water evaporates
and so removes heat from the gas and cools it. Air is drawn
through the condenser by a fan to assist evaporation. This air,
now warm and mixed with water vapour, is discharged upwards
to a vent on the roof. The system is not untypical, but at Pontiac

this vent was under a box-like structure with slatted sides – which also housed the intake vent of the air-conditioning system. So air full of water vapour from the evaporative condenser could be sucked into the duct which fed the air-conditioning unit, which then pumped it into the offices.

Guinea-pigs made to breathe an aerosol of water from the condenser developed pneumonia just like those placed in the offices. This suggested that some organism in the water had caused the outbreak of Pontiac fever but in 1968 CDC failed to find it. 'Pontiac was our Vietnam,' says Dr Michael Gregg, one of the epidemiologists who led the investigation. But they did not close the case. They stored blood samples from Pontiac patients in freezers. Eight years later when Gregg and his colleagues heard about Dr Fraser's findings at Philadelphia they noted certain similarities. When later they heard of McDade's break-through they put the blood samples from Pontiac through the IFA fluorescence test: over eighty-five per cent of the cases had antibody to *Legionella*.

They had also stored samples of lung from the dead guinea-pigs. When these were cultured, colonies of *Legionella* appeared. This proved that Pontiac fever was caused by the same organism as Legionnaires' disease. But Pontiac fever is less severe – no one died of it – and there are three other major differences. Legionnaires' disease is primarily a pneumonia but no one at Pontiac developed pneumonia. Secondly, Legionnaires' disease affects around five per cent of people exposed to it, whereas Pontiac fever affects ninety-five per cent or more. Thirdly, the incubation period – the interval between exposure to infection and the onset of symptoms – ranges from two to ten days in Legionnaires' disease but averaged only a day or two in Pontiac fever. Why the same bacterium can cause these two very different diseases is still a mystery, though it is under active investigation.

So *Legionella pneumophila* had been incriminated at Philadelphia and Pontiac, in both places *after* the event. To take any steps towards treatment, what CDC needed was a chance to identify *Legionella* in a new outbreak. It came at Burlington, Vermont, a city of 60,000 right up in the north-east near the Canadian border. This time the outbreak started in a hospital, the Vermont Medical Center. In the early summer of 1977 some patients in hospital for other diseases developed pneumonia. The hospital staff could find no causative micro-organism, but they had read about the newly-identified Legionnaires' disease, and so blood samples were sent to CDC on the off-chance that the Burlington patients might have it. The answer was yes.

By the time the news reached Burlington there were many more cases. Some had had no contact with the hospital, and had obviously caught the disease elsewhere in the city. Of the twelve who had caught the disease in hospital, four were in the dialysis unit for kidney disease, and two had had kidney transplants. The outbreak showed that *Legionella* prefers to strike people whose resistance is lowered by other causes such as transplants, kidney disease, and cancer.

The Burlington doctors, led by Dr Harry Beaty, treated the cases with a range of antibiotics. They found that one of them – erythromycin – was the most effective in keeping down the death rate, far more effective than penicillin. This was a vital discovery for the future. Erythromycin has remained the drug of choice against Legionnaires' disease to this day.

Of sixty-nine cases in Burlington, eleven died during the outbreak which went on for three months. CDC failed to find how the disease had been spread, or even whether it had a common source. But when blood tests were done on groups of healthy Burlington people they found that many carried antibody to *Legionella*. This suggested that the bacterium might be found in the natural environment as well as in man-made structures.

This possibility was confirmed by the next important outbreak which came in 1978 at Bloomington, Indiana, on the campus of the University of Indiana, which has 36,000 students. The outbreak centred on the Indiana Memorial Union, a large stone building, several storeys high, which houses student facilities and clubs and a hotel wing for visitors. Beginning in March 1978 the outbreak struck thirty-nine people, of whom thirty-five had spent at least one night in the hotel.

When a team from CDC arrived they investigated a cooling tower on top of the Union building. A cooling tower operates on the same principle as an evaporative condenser, but in a system where the circulating air is cooled by contact with cold water. The water heats up in the process. In order to cool it, it is pumped up to the top of the cooling tower to be sprayed down over slats which break it into droplets. These partially evaporate as they fall, losing heat, and are collected in a trough at the bottom. This cooled water is then recycled to the air-conditioning plant. To help the evaporation process a fan at the top of the tower draws a powerful current of air up through the slats, taking some of the droplets with it and dispersing them into the atmosphere.

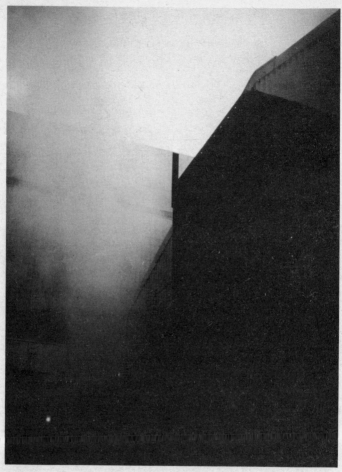

Another way Legionnaires' disease can spread: a cooling tower linked to an air conditioning system. It discharges water vapour containing Legionella pneumophila, *which is then breathed in by nearby humans.*

Had prevailing winds, blowing across the cooling tower at Bloomington, picked up droplets of infected water and carried them to the hotel wing below? This theory could not be proved, and anyhow the first cases had been in March before the air-conditioning was switched on. The investigators were left with a mystery, but they made one important new discovery. A stream runs through the campus alongside the Union building. Samples of water from it contained *Legionella;* and so did samples of earth from the nearby bank. This was the first proof that *Legionella* is able to live in nature as well as in man-made structures. Whether – and how – it got from the stream and up to the cooling tower a hundred yards away remains an open question.

The Bloomington outbreak went on until August 1978. In that same month another one started in Memphis, Tennessee, once again in a hospital. The Baptist Memorial Hospital is the largest private hospital in the world. Technicians in the pathology lab, run by Dr Richard Kelly, were among the first outside CDC to learn how to diagnose Legionnaires' Disease.

In August 1978 they did the IFA fluorescence test on a number of patients with pneumonia, and found antibody to *Legionella.* Because of the recent news from Bloomington Dr Kelly investigated the air-conditioning system. This is served by a large cooling tower on a roof on the west side of the hospital complex. He found no *Legionella* in it. But it so happened that on 8 August the main cooling tower had been put out of action because a flash flood had invaded the basement where the air-conditioning plant was located. To maintain air conditioning an auxiliary plant and cooling tower on the east side of the hospital had been brought into operation for a month. All thirty-nine cases around the hospital had been infected during that month. Dr Kelly took samples of water from the auxiliary tower, and injected them into guinea-pigs, as the first step in the CDC technique to see if the water contained *Legionella.* The guinea-pigs sickened and died; and their tissues were found to contain the bacterium.

Meanwhile investigators from CDC had been using a smoke generator to trace the air currents around the auxiliary tower. They found that one current could have carried infected water droplets up to the north-east wing to two air intakes. Most of the cases among patients occurred in the rooms supplied by these intakes. Another current spiralled down from the auxiliary cooling tower to the main hospital entrance below. Some staff and visitors who used this entrance developed Legionnaires' disease, as did four people who merely passed along the street beside it. The Memphis outbreak confirmed the evidence from Pontiac that Legionnaires' disease can be spread by air conditioning, but this was not the whole story, as events in Europe were soon to prove.

The first outbreak in Britain was investigated retrospectively. In Britain the function exercised by CDC is divided between two centres: the Communicable Diseases Surveillance Centre, at

Colindale in London, responsible for England and Wales; and the Communicable Diseases Unit, in Glasgow, to cover Scotland. The director of the Glasgow centre, Dr Dan Reid, was listening to the radio in his car in August 1976 when he heard the news of the Philadelphia outbreak. The circumstances, including summertime respiratory illness after a stay in a hotel, reminded him of a similar outbreak in Scotland three years before. On 24 July 1973 the control tower at Abbotsinch Airport, Glasgow, was informed that there was a seriously ill man on a plane returning from Spain with a load of 'package tourists'. An ambulance was ordered but by the time the plane landed the man was dead. Many others on board were ill – some were coughing. Within days nine had been taken to hospital, and two more men died of pneumonia.

When Dr Reid investigated, the full story was startling. There were 189 people on the ten-day tour. They had stayed in a new fourteen-storey hotel called the Rio Park in the seaside resort of Benidorm. Many had become ill in Benidorm – sixty-five per cent of them ill enough to go to bed during their stay or immediately on returning home. Of these fifty-one per cent had respiratory illness on top of gastro-intestinal disorders.

Dr Reid and the Spanish health authorities carried out extensive tests in Benidorm – on food and drink, and on the environment inside and outside the hotel. They looked for traces of insecticidal and other poisons as well as for micro-organisms. All their tests were negative, and so were those on the patients in Scotland. Dr Reid had to be content with storing clinical samples against some later development. Now here it was – in Philadelphia. As soon as Dr Reid heard of McDade's breakthrough in early 1977 he sent blood samples from the 1973 Scottish outbreak to Atlanta which identified the culprit as *Legionella*, and so confirmed his hunch that the Scottish tourists had indeed caught Legionnaires' disease in Spain. The mode of spread remained a mystery: the Rio Park hotel had not got air conditioning. Eventually cultures of *Legionella*, and samples of blood sera known to contain antibody to it, were sent to the Public Health Laboratory Service in Britain, so that British labs could now take an active part in diagnosing the disease. Seven PHLS labs were equipped in this way, one of them at Oxford.

In January 1979 a fifty-four-year-old woman in the Churchill Hospital in Oxford developed pneumonia. She was in the Renal Transplant Unit and was just recovering from a kidney transplant operation. Immediately after such an operation patients are nursed in one of six isolation rooms. In this case the woman was in Room Six. Her pneumonia was so serious that she had to be kept alive by artificial ventilation. Clinical samples were tested in the Oxford PHLS lab for pneumonia-causing organisms. On slides of bronchial material from her lung they found *Legionella*. She was given erythromycin and recovered.

It seemed likely that she had caught the infection in Room Six where she had spent ten days. A team led by Dr John Tobin examined the room. They scraped paint from the walls, dust from the ventilation grills, and in the adjoining bathroom they took swabs from the taps and waste-pipe of the sink, and from the water-closet. In none of these samples did they find any trace of *Legionella*.

Mindful of the reports from the United States, they then examined the air-conditioning plant which was in a room on the roof of the Renal Unit. Here they opened the compartment in which air flowed through filter bags down to the isolation rooms below. They put a cage of guinea-pigs inside, but these did not get ill: they actually grew fat. So the source of the infection remained a mystery.

Six months later another woman at the Churchill Hospital who had had a kidney transplant developed Legionnaires' disease. She too had been in Room Six. Dr Tobin's team did the environmental tests all over again, but this time they also took samples of water from the shower apparatus in the bathroom – from the mixing assembly and the side-arms. In these at last they found *Legionella*. When material from here was injected into guinea-pigs they got fever and died; and *Legionella* was isolated from their tissues.

In the plant room on the roof there are also two tanks supplying water to the Renal Unit. No *Legionella* was found in the water but as a precaution each tank was emptied and scrubbed, then refilled with water to which chlorine was added. This was flushed through the system before being replaced with ordinary water. In addition all the showers were taken out of service. Since then there have been no further cases of the disease in the Renal Unit.

The discovery that *Legionella* can lurk in ordinary tap-water systems gave a dramatic new slant to its potential threat. Confirmation was not long in coming. Later in 1979 there was an outbreak of Legionnaires' disease among a party of golfers who had stayed in a hotel at Corby, an industrial town in Northamptonshire. There were only four cases, none fatal, but the Oxford team, together with Dr Christopher Bartlett, consultant epidemiologist at Colindale, were called in to investigate.

There was no air conditioning in the hotel but they found *Legionella* in the hot and cold water systems and in the cold-water storage tank. They found none in the mains water supply. The installation of a continuous chlorination plant, which keeps the chlorine level in the cold water system around one or two parts per million, has kept the hotel free of further cases.

The Communicable Diseases Control Centre at Colindale is notified of cases of infectious disease from all over England. In the summer of 1980 Dr Bartlett was able to spot an outbreak of Legionnaires' disease by collating reports about a number of cases in different parts of the country. They showed a common factor: they had all just returned from a holiday in Spain. Even more astonishing, they had all stayed at the Rio Park in Benidorm, the hotel implicated in the Scottish outbreak of 1973. Dr Bartlett went to Benidorm by agreement with the Spanish authorities. There is no air-conditioning plant in the Rio Park, but when they tested the tap water they found *Legionella*, notably in a hand-shower set over the basin in the hairdressing salon, and in some of the bedroom showers.

That same year, 1980, there was a second important outbreak in Britain – in the General Hospital at Kingston-upon-Thames just outside London. One of the pathology staff at Kingston was Dr Sue Fisher-Hoch who had worked with Dr Tobin on the Oxford cases. At Kingston she trained lab technicians to look for *Legionella* in routine clinical samples, and in March 1980 it turned up in a serum sample.

The victim was a twenty-year-old medical student who had been doing vacation work as a cleaner in one of the hospital's many buildings – a seven-storey block opened in 1976. It contains surgical, medical, and paediatric wards, some of which look out onto an internal courtyard. Dr Fisher-Hoch sounded a first discreet alarm – one such case was not an outbreak. But in mid-May two more cases were diagnosed in hospital patients over one weekend. Both were in the new block. Dr Bartlett and Dr Tobin were called in, and an intensive investigation began.

The new block had an air-conditioning system but guinea-pigs placed in the distribution ducts did not get sick even after a month's exposure. Samples of water from the cooling tower on the roof did contain *Legionella*, so they drained the tower at the end of May, and cleansed it with water containing fifty parts per million of chlorine – a truly massive dose: swimming pools are kept sterile with three parts per million!

Samples of water taken from taps and showers in the new block contained enough *Legionella* to kill guinea-pigs; and it was also found in some of the older hospital buildings though, mysteriously, no one got infected in those. Perhaps the concentration of *Legionella* in the new block was greater – and more lethal? Finally, they checked the mains water-supply and even the Water Board's reservoirs – and found nothing.

While the investigation was going on, in June and July, three more cases occurred, two of them fatal. These fuelled a hysterical campaign in the local and national media over the persistence of this 'mystery killer disease'. The hospital authorities were accused of covering up the true facts – an irony since it was only Dr Fisher-Hoch's unusual vigilance which had spotted the outbreak in the first place. Unfortunately some of the staff, mostly foreign ancillary workers, began to panic. One trade union demanded the right to investigate how the outbreak was being managed, and at least one union official called for the hospital to be closed.

In mid-July, at a special meeting, this option was seriously considered, but it was argued that to close the hospital would kill more patients than were likely to die from Legionnaires' disease. To find alternative accommodation for hundreds of patients would prove very difficult; they would have to be sent home, and many might die for lack of suitable treatment. Scientific argument, and the common sense of most of the staff, prevented closure, and control of the outbreak was achieved with the hospital working normally.

A continuous chlorination plant was installed and by the end of July monitoring of water outlets throughout the hospital showed that a suitable level of chlorine – between one and two parts per million – was being maintained in the cold-water system. More importantly, no *Legionella* could be found in it. The hot-water system proved more difficult because chlorine blows off as the temperature rises, and at 45°C – the average in the hospital's hot taps – the chlorine level was not high enough to kill *Legionella*. So in August they raised the temperature to between 55 and 60°C, quite enough to kill all *Legionella*, but also enough to scald incautious patients! Warning notices had to be posted to prevent accidents. There remained the cooling tower – an urgent problem given the result of wind studies done to see whether water droplets could have carried infection. These showed that, with the wind in a certain quarter, droplets could drift across the roof and be sucked down into the courtyard well and into open windows of the wards on the top floor – precisely where most of the Legionnaires' disease cases had been.

The cooling tower stayed free of *Legionella* for some weeks, after the initial treatment in May, but it was found again at the end of July: water in the tower was warm enough to blow off the sterilising chlorine, and as no reliable method of maintaining the chlorine level could be devised, the tower was taken out of service for good in November. But by then there were no further cases in the hospital – the last had been in mid-July: for the first time in Britain an outbreak of Legionnaires' disease had been identified and brought under control while it was in progress. It was a practical success, but one which once again left in doubt the mode of spread. The first case at Kingston had occurred in March, before the air-conditioning system with its cooling tower came into operation, and must therefore have been infected from another source, probably the tap water. British experts were confirmed in their view that this is the primary source, and that air-conditioning systems are secondary but American epidemiologists remain sceptical about the significance of these British findings. If the British are right, how can tap water, in the absence of air-conditioning plants, give you the disease? Probably not by drinking it but by inhaling a fine aerosol such as can be produced by shower heads. This theory is being investigated at centres in Britain and at the University of Vermont in the USA.

Also being investigated are better methods of preventing the build-up of *Legionella* in cooling towers and evaporative condensers. These are usually dosed with disinfectants to kill algae, fungi, and slime-forming bacteria, and if this is done regularly the disinfectants should also kill *Legionella*. For tap-water systems, more reliable and cheaper methods of control are under study. Prolonged use of high levels of chlorine will corrode metal pipes, and to keep hot water around the necessary 55°C is costly: and there is the danger of scalding.

Even if much research remains to be done on such problems, enough is already known to put the threat posed by *Legionella* in perspective. Legionnaires' disease has now been reported from most countries of the world where techniques of identification are available. In Britain there is a steady trickle of sporadic cases, but outbreaks occur only very occasionally, and usually during the summer months. About 1000 cases a year are admitted to hospital, but with the specific treatment available only about 100 die of the disease. By comparison, 55,000 people a year die of other types of pneumonia.

On the other hand epidemiologists like Dr Fraser point to the fact that in the United States there are three million cases of pneumonia a year, and that in one million the cause is unknown. He believes there is a possibility that some of these cases may be caused by *Legionella* – like organisms. Already four other species of *Legionella* itself have been discovered, and there may be more to come. McDade's discovery of a whole new genus of organisms has shown scientists that surprises are still possible in the mysterious world of micro-organisms.

So the medical detective's work is exceedingly complicated. It requires expert knowledge from many fields. The international nature of medical research is enormously beneficial. There have been successes. Through the efforts of the World Health Organisation (WHO) the smallpox virus, at least in its most deadly form, is now extinct – as dead as that other famous organism, the dodo. But there have also been failures. The major cancers have scarcely been touched by the search for cures (although there have been successes in the minor ones) neither has heart disease. The more that environmental factors, such as stress, eating habits and pollution, come into the picture, the more obscure and difficult it becomes.

Money helps. Not just money for research; in fact President Nixon's mammoth anti-cancer campaign, in which millions of dollars were poured into the problem, was a failure. It is the wealth of the community which matters. Rich countries see very few cases of the typhoid and cholera which rampage through poorer countries, and virtually none of the starvation-related diseases such as marasmus and kwashiorkor. In the 1930s it was money spent on cleaner living conditions that brought down the level of tuberculosis so dramatically, not the drugs which were introduced later.

Third World countries naturally, therefore, come off worst in the health stakes. They suffer from many diseases, such as malaria or onchocerciasis (African river blindness), which are perfectly treatable and preventable but remain endemic. Western methods often simply do not work – for political and even cultural reasons. A typical example is bilharzia (schistosomiasis). The case against the disease was relatively easy to solve; the real problems lie elsewhere.

8 The Qualyub Project

Edward Goldwyn

In recent years there has been increasing interest in Arab science. With the money that oil brings, new universities have been set up in Syria and Saudi Arabia specifically to study the science of the medieval Arab world, its mathematics, astronomy and medicine. New university laboratories are expanding in the Middle East, and a generation of modern Arab scientists is being created.

It is argued that the new Arab science should be different from that which grew up in Europe. The Koran specifically commands that man contemplate the world and use the knowledge he so gains for the benefit of all: it is wrong to grow the tree of scientific understanding in a lopsided way. That is, it would be against Arab tradition to specialise to any great extent. The question being debated in *Nature* and the *New Scientist,* and at many international conferences, is whether the new Arab science will be different from the science of the West. It was to explore that that we went to Egypt. For Egypt has the strongest scientific tradition of all Muslim countries. It has eight major universities and more scientists and engineers graduate from there than from the rest of the Arab world.

Egypt is poor – and there is not much of it. At first glance a map shows it to look bigger than France – but almost all Egyptian life is confined to a narrow track of green leaves and black earth winding across a glaring yellow desert. On the margin of this ten-mile-wide country, a hundred paces carries you from the open heat of eye-searing sandy light into shade on black earth, under palms, surrounded by crops, irrigation canals and bright-eyed, friendly, cheerful poverty. The Delta too has these sharp edges – but here the silt of centuries has created an unlimited flatness that feels like Holland.

Egypt is the Nile – and for millennia the Water Authority has managed its waters with an extraordinarily careful organisation. In Biblical times the Bahr Yousef canal carried water 200 miles to make the Fayoum depression, which would otherwise have been arid, the richest part of the old Pharaonic kingdom. For millennia almost all of the Nile's water has been taken into canals. It was, and still is, used to flood field after field, according to strict and detailed cycles. Each farmer knows by heart which three days in each fortnight his ditches will be filled, and he chooses accordingly his time to plant, to weed and to harvest. It is said that Egyptian science grew from a need to predict the time and weight of the annual Nile flood.

The construction of the high dam at Aswan, opened in 1971, began major changes in Egypt, and caused three problems in particular which now have high priority. The National Research Council has set major teams to work on them. The first is a problem that seems simple but isn't. The Egyptians need something to build with: up to the present they have used bricks. The Nile outside Cairo looks like nineteenth-century Manchester. Rows and rows of high chimneys, about a quarter of a mile apart for miles on end, pour out never-ending black smoke as the kilns bake Egypt's rich earth into building bricks. In the days before the Aswan dam the dug-out earth was made good with silt. Now, as the earth is used it is leaving flooded, unreplenished land at an alarming rate: land impossible to farm. For some years it has been announced officially that brick-making must stop – but since no substitute has been found, it has to go on.

The second problem that follows the damming of the Nile is drainage. Now that the land is irrigated the whole year round, it is not drying out as it used to. The water table has risen to just a few inches below the surface. The land is becoming infertile because the salts are not being carried away. The waterlogged ground also means large buildings (including the Pyramids) are in danger of sinking. The solution is to build a new network of drainage canals to get the salted water down to the sea. The challenge is how to integrate them into the existing system – and how to raise the huge sum of money to pay for them.

The third problem is a disease called Schistosomiasis, which is caused by a parasite that lives in the water. It has been known in Egypt for 3000 years: a mummy has been found with ova of the parasite, and on the writings in the pyramid of Lahun a hieroglyph shows a penis passing blood – a common symptom of the disease. But since the damming of the Nile it has become more prevalent and widespread. It is transmitted by snails and now – as the ditches are no longer baked hard-dry in the hot sun – the snails are spreading to new areas in increased numbers.

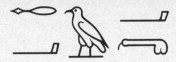

Egyptian hieroglyph for the word âaâ, *generally taken to mean haematuria, a symptom of schistosomiasis.*

Schistosomiasis, sometimes called Bilharzia, is not only an Egyptian problem. It is the world's second most common disease; one in twelve suffer from it. Napoleon's troops caught it when they conquered Egypt, and it infected many British soldiers in the Second World War.

Nowadays there is a big international effort to cure this disease. Although it occurs in other parts of the world, most of the experimental fieldwork is concentrated in Egypt – and the Egyptian government give their Schistosomiasis scientists considerable priority.

The premier field station for this study is in an old colonial country house in the small town of Qualyub that lies about an hour's drive beyond the slums of Cairo, north along the edge of the Nile, past the dhows and the brick chimneys on the riverbank. For more than twenty years there has been continuous work here, surveying the health of the villagers, surveying the disease, the snails, assessing the effectiveness of all the different attempts to prevent the disease – which until recently had little success. The research project is well staffed and equipped, and its director is a man of considerable skill. It was through him, in coming to understand his ambitions, his priorities and how he is making them happen, that we came to see there *was* something tangibly different about Arab science.

Dr Muhammed el Alamy, the director of the Qualyub project, is open in his reactions, firm in his opinions and with a ready smile. He is proud of Egypt and her culture. He is religious, and attends the Mosque on Friday whenever he can. He has lived in Egypt most of his life, apart from a postgraduate degree taken in the USA.

Dr Alamy says that besides the goal of controlling Schistosomiasis, his deeper ambition is to train the young doctors who work for him to become good scientists doing prestigious work of their own – but to train them in such a way that they choose to do their work in Egypt, instead of being lured away by the glamour of the USA, or else driven away because they can't cope with the

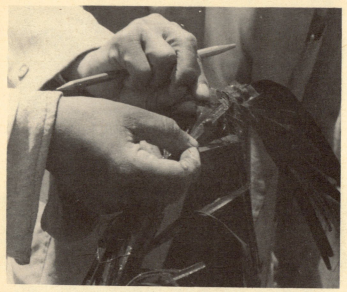

Freshwater snails of the kind that act as transmitters of schistosomiasis.

awful difficulties of doing research in Egypt. These difficulties were only slowly to become apparent to us.

Schistosomiasis is caused by wormlike parasites that come from another infected person; but the disease is only infective if it comes via one kind of water snail. The worms are about ½″ long and live in the veins around the human gut and bladder. There are two varieties of the disease, which are caused by worms that look similar, but are of different species. The worms lay eggs and these pass out of the human in the urine for one species of the worm (*haematobium*) and in the feces for the second (*mansoni*).

If an egg falls into water during urination or defecation it hatches within minutes. Micracidia emerge from the eggs and swim through the water: each looks like a piece of dust caught in the sunlight. It will live for six to seventy-two hours. It is not infective to humans – it only has the capacity to infect one particular species of snail. It can swim quite rapidly, covering about six inches in two or three minutes. A micracidium is actively attracted by the odour of a snail, and, if it finds the snail, burrows into it.

Nothing seems noticeably different about the snail for a

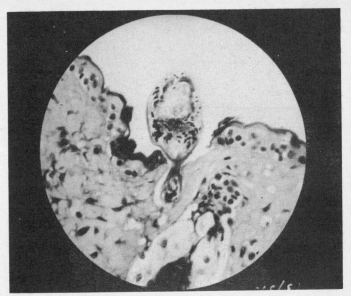

Microscopic view of a cercaria penetrating the skin.

month or so – but then a startling change takes place. The snail becomes a factory which manufactures copies of the parasite. It releases clouds of them each day into the water. A snail can live for nine months, releasing 2000 parasites a day. The parasites are now in a new form, a millimetre or so long, called cercariae. It is this form that is infective to humans. The cercariae are attracted by the heat of a person's skin, or failing that by the light. They swim actively in the water at midday; they are ready at the time when most people use the water; they take as little as four minutes to penetrate a person's skin; and once into the bloodstream they are carried to the liver.

There over a period of eight weeks, they grow into mature male and female worms and then each searches for a mate. The female climbs inside the male, where she lives for the rest of her life. The male with the female inside crawls out to the veins around the bladder or gut, and there they live for twenty years, releasing one egg every six minutes.

It is the eggs, not the worms, that do the damage. It is a mixture of mechanical damage, as the spiky hard eggs get stuck in the body's organs, and chronic inflammation, as the immune

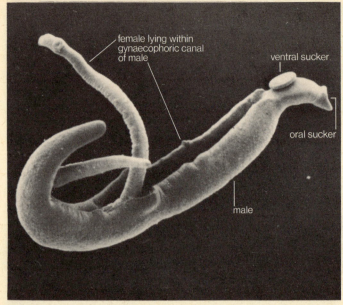

female lying within
gynaecophoric canal
of male

ventral sucker

oral sucker

male

Mature female worm inside the male.

system reacts against them. One of the first symptoms is usually blood in the urine, caused by the eggs bursting through the bladder wall. The progress of the disease is not predictable. Some people live without symptoms, others die within a year. For many, the eggs slowly destroy the liver or the kidney, causing twenty years of ill health and an early death.

It was in 1857 at a Cairo hospital (that is still there) that a young German doctor Theodor Bilharz (the disease is still often called Bilharzia) discovered the worms and eggs in a series of post mortems. He believed but had no proof that the victims had caught the parasites from the water. Indeed the Pharaohs of ancient Egypt also believed that, and related the disease to human excreta in the water. One had engraved on the wall of his tomb in a list of his good deeds: 'I never fouled the water.'

It was in 1915 that the full lifecycle and the importance of the snail was worked out. It was done by the British in Egypt picking up on Japanese work that had shown mice exposed to water con-

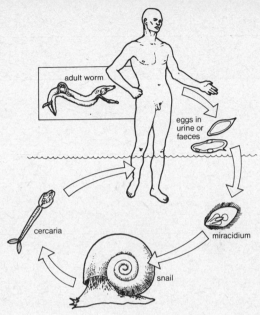

The life cycle of the schistosome.

taining cercarie became ill. The work was done in order to find ways to protect the British army in Egypt.

It looks at first glance as though it ought to be relatively easy to break the cycle, and so wipe out the disease. Various possible strategies suggest themselves: to keep eggs out of the water (by building latrines); or to remove all the snails (with poison); or to prevent people being infected (by educating them not to go into the water), or to prevent eggs being excreted by humans (by poisoning the worms in the veins).

However up till now there has been little impact on the disease outside China. There, whole provinces were mobilised to fill the old ditches and to build new ones. They kept the canals free of weed and had regular snail hunts. These measures applied with their discipline and thoroughness led to huge improvements in the 1950s and 60s.

Drugs have been tried with some success for decades, but until very recently the drugs have had such serious side effects that it has not been possible to use them widely. Drugs which could kill the worm while still in the veins were found, but they were extremely toxic. Tartar emetic was used and it had to be injected directly into the bloodstream, twelve times over a few weeks. It was fifty per cent effective but a person had to be in good health to stand its poisonous action on the liver. Since the Sixties and Seventies oxamniquine and metrifiamate have become available, but still a patient had to be relatively fit to take them. More recently, a new drug called biltricide has proved effective on all species of Bilharzias. It is given by mouth in a single dose, is well tolerated by patients and is promising.

Although there have been massive eradication attempts, poisoning snails has not worked as a strategy, except for a few cases with special geography, where there is a single water source. It was not at first realised how fast they could multiply and repopulate the canals. Nevertheless there have been continual attempts to improve the poisons, and techniques and many campaigns are still active.

It costs a great deal in manpower and chemicals. Complex machinery is used to pump the chemicals in, and there are teams of workers along each canal measuring poison concentration – for the permitted range is small. It must be less than that which makes the water lethal to fish and man – and yet high enough to kill the snails.

The first successful control came only in 1969. It was decided to experiment with a two-pronged attack to achieve not eradication but control. The area selected was the Fayoum. It is a large depression, about the size of Kent, to one side of the Nile about sixty miles south-west of Cairo. It is the area the Pharaohs made extremely rich, and today it is still fed by one huge canal – the Bahr Youssef – that they built. By putting the snail poison into this canal they could treat the whole region. It takes four days for the poison to go through the district. They have to treat on six separate days each time, so that each irrigation ditch is treated as it takes its turn in the cycle. The chemicals cost £1 million a year and it takes an army of 250 men on bicycles to police all the canals. They make snail population surveys and call up a truck or a team of hand sprayers to mop up any focus of snails they find. Attacking snails was prong one, prong two of the control strategy was to reduce the egg output from the humans.

Because the side effects of the drug were so serious people couldn't be given the drug if they were not really ill with Schistosomiasis. They couldn't simply treat everybody, which would have been cheap and easy. All the population, over one million,

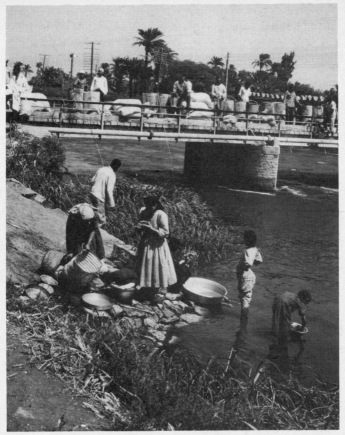

Egyptian workers lower snail poison into the water of a canal from a bridge.

were persuaded to provide a sample of urine and faeces. It was found that about half of them were infected. They all had to be examined by a doctor. Eighty per cent were well enough to be treated, and almost all of them were.

The result is that now the waters of the Fayoum are safe. It's not a cure – if the snail poisoning or the screening and treatment of the people stopped – then enough eggs and snails would meet to make the water infective again. It's not cheap either. To set up medical services capable of examining everyone by a doctor, as well as organising the poisoning, is more than Egypt – or any Third World country – can afford except as a special demonstration project. And that is why the work at Qualyub is so important, for they are doing the field trial of a new drug that could slash the cost of controlling the disease.

In the last few years the Beyer company has developed a new drug, Praziquantel. It is completely effective in killing the parasite, and so far has shown no side effects. If this finding is borne out by the Qualyub trial, then it can be used to treat anybody who agrees to take it – with no examination necessary. People will not only be cured but the cycle will be broken at costs a Third World country, granted some aid, can afford.

The drug has been through its hospital in-patient trials (thirty people) and its doctor-supervised clinical trials (a few hundred). Now it is Dr Muhammed el Alamy's task at Qualyub to try it in the field under conditions like those under which it will be used. His problems are enormous. The drug is being given to 20,000 people and their health compared to that of 20,000 not receiving the drug. All 40,000 have full medical check-ups as well as tests for eggs before the trial. Those infected, in the experimental group, have to be persuaded to take the treatment. They are all rechecked after three months and after one year. One fifth of a million samples of urine and feces will have to be processed and examined under microscopes.

The project staff have to make detailed maps of each village, interview each household to compile their own up-to-date census.

The value of the trial depends as much on the sense of responsibility and care among very junior staff and consistent careful administration as it does on scientific measurement. In that Alamy faces the particular problems of the Third World: transient politicians and civil servants, changing policies, very low wages and above all a brain drain.

Egypt trains more Arabic speaking scientists and technicians than all the Arab nations taken together. But the Kuwaitis and the Saudis want them for their new hospitals and universities. Egypt is poor: salaries are five to ten times higher in the Gulf. Egyptians who go (officially for two years, but many seem to stay longer) earn enough to buy on their return a house, a car, an education for their children and still have savings to live on. It is Egypt's loss and often quite unnecessary for the patron country anyway. The most distinguished professors of parasitology at a Cairo university are almost continuously in Kuwait teaching rich men's sons who are taking biology degrees at university as a status symbol. Most of their students will never do anything with their degrees, but will inherit their fathers' businesses, which have no connections with parasites, in a country which does not have Schistosomiasis anyway.

The brain drain is also severe in the case of technicians who in Egypt earn trivial salaries, set nationally by Ministry of Health regulations. At some prestigious laboratories in Cairo we were told that research was severely hampered because many technicians hurried through their work, often inventing results to be away by twelve o'clock. We were told they had to leave by twelve to get to their second job. The Ministry pays technicians about £30 a month. It's low because in Egypt all trained people are promised they will get a government job and there is overmanning. It's unofficially recognised that most will need a second job and a blind eye is turned if they go early. Ministry technicians do not choose where they'll work, they are allocated to their job. So generally there isn't a responsible attitude towards accuracy.

Alamy is very dependent on his junior staff – not only technicians but the humbly-paid workers who deal with the villagers. Finding the right villager and finding him or her again and again takes a lot of commitment. And then they have to persuade and cajole them to hand over specimens. The staff have to be vigilant to ensure they are getting a specimen from all the proper people – and that someone behind the scenes has not filled all the family's pots personally, just to keep the project staff happy and save the bother of chasing off to find the people who forgot when they went off at sunrise to work in the fields. And as the hundreds of samples a day go through the testing there are many, many steps at which a mistake could be made, sample numbers miscopied or results invented.

Alamy's relationship to his staff, and the atmosphere in the laboratories, are difficult to convey. There is fear and love. There is remarkable cleanliness. The floors are swept, everyone wears fresh lab coats or overalls. You can feel the effort to keep the old buildings and gardens neat, in marked contrast with the streets outside, which are littered with cans and bits of paper. Alamy will make a point of bending down himself to pick up something from the floor when a nod from him would bring a houseboy to do it. He knows his staff see, and that action communicates more strongly than words.

Alamy trains his technicians carefully. He gets them directly from school (so they have not learned a slap-happy attitude), and they spend months learning the techniques. When counting eggs in real samples they find their pay is linked to a fierce quality-

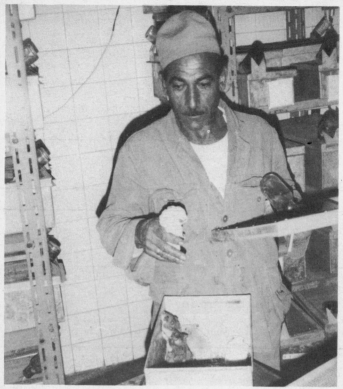

One of Dr El-Alamy's research staff at work.

control system. The samples are coded by number – quite a few
being repeat samples from the same patients – and a technician
doesn't know if he is in fact re-checking a test done by him or
another person earlier in the day. Only Alamy and the senior
technician know that. If a person's work is accurate he will take
home double pay. If not, he won't.

But beside coercion there is concern. By a well-placed tele-
phone call, Alamy will see that their husbands, wives and parents
will get good medical treatment. He will continue to keep in
touch so the hospital know that someone in a high place is
watching this case and that's important in Cairo. He knows his
staff well enough to find out if a period of being late or in-
accurate is due to trouble at home, and he is generous in sending
people off to deal with what is worrying them.

He says: 'When anyone has a problem he comes to me. He conveys to me his problem and I take care of that. I always try to satisfy my people. You can't get the brain of someone who is worried. So you let them relax and they will give you what you want.'

Near the top of the hierarchy of project staff are the four doctors. They are all aged about thirty, and half have post-graduate degrees. These people Alamy sees as critically important. They will become the next generation of Egypt's senior scientists. It is on them that his deepest ambitions for Egyptian science will be fulfilled. But the brain drain operates even more temptingly on doctors than on technicians.

After graduation doctors must remain in Egypt for a com-pulsory period of time. After that they could earn a fortune in the oil-rich Gulf states. During this compulsory period Alamy can give not much more than the government wage of £50 a month, and they can't manage on that. So most doctors in government employment have a private practice as well. Alamy encourages this, and actively helps them to set up as general practitioners in the small towns of the Delta, and he does this for two reasons besides the money they will earn.

Firstly, he says their medicine will be constantly expanded. Dealing only with 'schisto' for years can make one too special-ised a doctor; and, secondly, he wants them to evolve an under-standing and compassion for the peasant people of Egypt. When that happens, Alamy says, 'he will be more stuck to this earth, and so he will hesitate to go or be taken by the Saudis or Kuwaitis or those people who have more money. This is my idea, and it has succeeded.'

Alamy's relationship with his senior staff is different from that which we find familiar in the West. In Egypt seniority commands many signs of respect. Alamy's doctors would not smoke nor cross their legs in his presence, and only sit if he invited them to. They would not contradict him – and would think carefully before venturing a point of view different from his. They would always refer to him formally as 'Dr Alamy' and never be more familiar. Yet these were doctors with years of experience and postgraduate degrees. When one doctor was asked, 'could you never think of calling him Muhammed?' she was overcome with embarrassment and laughter and said: 'Never – no – of course not.'

He has much more power over their lives than he would in the West. He is their patron. Primarily it is through him they get the

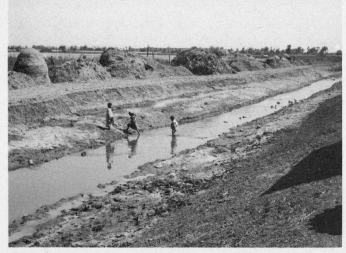

Barefoot children paddle in one of the canals of Lower Egypt.

chance for promotion or transfer to another job within the Ministry. Only through his arranging it will they go on post-graduate courses in Egypt, the USA or Europe. Once he has accepted them onto his staff they expect him to look after their careers, just as he sees it as his responsibility and obligation to help them forward – much as a father would act for his children. They in return treat him like a father, bow to his authority with respect and follow the career he designs for them.

While making the film we found it increasingly hard to re-concile Alamy's ambition to make his staff into inquisitive scientists, able to manage research projects on their own, with his allowing them to accept such an obedient role. Broadly speaking, he did little to encourage them to be critical and independent. That conflict was to become acute when we set out – simply, so it seemed – to make a visit with the doctors to a village to plan the filming there.

The journey was by minibus, all the staff and ourselves talking with enthusiasm and gusto as we trucked along earth roads raising a cloud of dust that enveloped donkey carts and the occasional old dented and groaning bus or lorry.

The village we arrived at was romantic in the extreme. Mud huts lined the narrow streets. There were huge bundles of stalks stored on the flat roofs ready to be used for fuel. Chickens, children and dogs played on the baked earth streets among the women sitting in groups, trading vegetables or chatting. Black hoods, glittering earrings, bright dresses. After a surprising number of near misses, we pulled up at the village clinic and we went in.

We knew that in the villages the men and women spend many hours each day standing in the water. The men walk along the canals and stand ankle-deep in the water, sowing seeds and weeding. The women stand in the water to wash clothes and cooking pots. The children swim in the hot midday sun. The adults wash themselves in the water.

We asked the doctors to come with us and show us where was best to see the people in the water and we would choose places to film. To our amazement they said they had never been out beyond the clinic porch. In fact, they had shoes entirely unsuited to the puddles of mud and muck of the street. The women wore high heels – the men thin soled, low cut, highly polished shoes. Alamy had said that they as research workers should have the patients come in for examination. This meant that, as a rule they had no reason to go out of the clinic and so they didn't. But they said of course they would be delighted to come and help us: Alamy had instructed them to help us in any way they could. They seemed hurt to see so many people they knew in the water. When we asked the villagers why they didn't avoid contact with the water, the doctors interpreted as the villagers explained.

The farmers said that for their work they had to operate Archimedes screws to lift water from field to field and construct small mud dams to divert the water. And as many of them were hired very cheaply by the day, clearly the owner of the land wasn't going to provide expensive new equipment. And some said that anyway they were not totally convinced the water was that dangerous – they'd been standing in it for years, like their fathers before them.

The women said that, although there was a tap with clean water in the village, they used the canals because in the canal their soap lathered better. At the canal, they said, they could enjoy the conversation. Also you didn't have to carry water; the suds moved off with the flow of the stream, and water for rinsing moved to you. If you carried water home from the tap to wash with, you would have to carry it out of the village afterwards to be rid of it, for there was nowhere at home to pour it away. If they threw it into the street it would create dangerous pools of mud for the children and animals to slip about in. They said that carrying the families' drinking water – which they did get from the tap – was burden enough. And they said with emphasis that with the work at home, the cooking, looking after the children, the goats, the camels and taking their produce to sell at market, they had no time or energy to carry a lot more water about.

The doctors were emotionally wrung out by what we had involved them in. Although they knew it already in an abstract way, they were being confronted with the very people they had met inside the clinic, whom they had often told to beware of the water and who had probably said the equivalent of, 'Yes, doctor, of course, doctor.'

One of the doctors said: 'I think it was a very good experience for me. I only used to watch people from the windows of the bus. When they came to our clinic I just instructed them not to go into the water and to avoid it. But it is a major problem to avoid it because it's their work. I couldn't realise this without seeing them working in the water.'

We were in a conflict. It seemed to us that the obedience that an Egyptian staff give to their principal was at odds with our concept of the necessity of developing the questioning and critical abilities of a scientist. We asked Alamy whether there wasn't a contradiction in his ambition for his doctors and the obedience he expected from them. Weren't his staff too afraid to develop their own ideas? His response was polite but firm.

'I think you look to this scenery from a different angle than we. This is our culture, you see. We are accustomed to look to our fathers and to our teachers with respect, with more than respect. And these young ladies and gentlemen whom you have seen either in the field or in the lab, they consider me as their teacher and their elder brother or father. That is why they behave this way. This is our culture; this is the normal way of behaviour. It is different from yours, and you are measuring me with your measure. If I go to London I may find something absolutely wrong, and you consider it normal. So you see, it is a difference of culture.'

Alamy had very good and practical reasons for maintaining the traditional Egyptian pattern. For his goal was not only to create good scientists and project leaders – but ones who will choose to stay in Egypt. To do that they must know how to operate the Egyptian way. To give them an abrasive, critical attitude would probably carry them permanently to the USA. So he tries to show them how to make good science work within the Egyptian culture: to teach them all the subtleties needed to succeed against the problems of a rapidly changing, too-powerful bureaucracy, of little money, low wages, of difficulties in getting equipment – in short, all the problems that make science so difficult in the Third World.

We came to feel the Egyptian science we saw *was* different from that in the West. It is very different from our idealised vision of an environment to encourage the abrasive free-thinking of an Einstein or a Crick. But what we experienced was subtle. It was finely tuned to bring the benefits of knowledge to the people.

And that is what the Koran says knowledge should be used for.

Maybe the new financial power behind scientists in Islam, especially medical scientists, will bring a new burgeoning of the old, medieval, Arab successes. But many have doubts. Most of the money, at present, is used to purchase high technology medicine from the West. When a strong, non-science-based ideology, like Communism or Islam or Catholicism before Luther, takes over a culture not much progress is made in science. No matter how much importance it is given, priorities get mixed up. In Soviet agriculture it led to Lysenkoism, after which thousands and possibly millions starved. In China, it was the cultural revolution and the wholesale destruction of laboratories by the Red Guards.

But Chinese science was not destroyed. China's problems have been related almost entirely to the size of her population. Control over food supplies, control over the devastation caused by natural disasters, control over disease have been central to Maoist thinking. And Western ideas and methods have not been rejected in the process – as they were in the Soviet Union. So, the last of our medical detective stories involves the combining of Western and Oriental science in an astonishingly successful campaign. It shows the art of medical science at its very best.

9 The Cancer Detectives of Lin Xian

Edward Goldwyn

A young schoolgirl sings to a crowd of peasants in a cold but bright sunlit Monday lunchbreak. She sings with enthusiasm and much expression. Her words are:

> Early discovery
> is very important.
> Take a balloon test.
> It's really important
> that you have regular check-ups
> for oesophageal cancer.
> Early discovery!
> The earlier it's found
> the better the cure.'

She is part of the campaign in Nan Yo, a production brigade village in the Lin Xian valley of Central China – a campaign organised by their barefoot doctor. He is responsible for wall posters and for the broadcasts over the village loudspeaker system, which exhort the people as they eat their evening meal in the last daylight to take the necessary steps to avoid cancer. He will visit and give a 'serious talk' to anyone he suspects is not taking the precautions he publicises.

Such campaigns are in progress in all the many small white-painted villages that are spread over the flat valley floor. On one side rise the flat-topped Taihang Mountains. On the other, the rolling hills separating this valley from the great central plain that stretches 300 miles to the sea.

This campaign is the first major Chinese experiment designed to eradicate cancer using the same techniques that were used so successfully in the past to wipe out their previous major diseases. But there is a difference. In the previous diseases they conquered – malaria, TB, hookworm, and so on – the causes were clear, and people could be told what to avoid. The fundamental

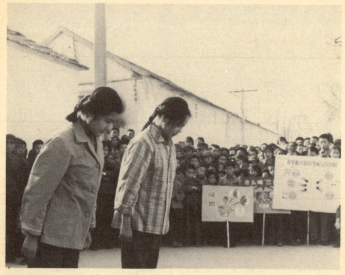

A village concert: girls sing about the symptoms of cancer and encourage people to seek early help.

problem with cancer is that its causes are largely unknown and certainly complex.

The inhabitants of the Lin Xian valley have been at the mercy of cancer of the oesophagus for centuries (there is a reference to it in writing from 2000 years ago). One in ten die of it, 100 times more than is normal. At one end of the valley the rate rises so that, in a area only twenty miles square, one in four people die of this cancer. Outwards from the valley, in concentric belts, the incidence of the cancer steadily decreases – until at about 300 miles it approaches normal levels. It is just cancer of the oesophagus that is so common, other cancers occur in their usual pattern.

Lin Xian seemed to be a unique experiment of nature in which scientists could begin research into cancer prevention. If they could find out what was special about this area, by comparing it with other areas, the cause of this particular cancer might be revealed.

A team of scientists was created by bringing epidemiologists, virologists, chemists and geologists from Peking and Chengchou (the capital city of the Honan province) to join the pathologists and surgeons of the local hospitals. They began their work in

1958. They were not expecting to find a single cause of the cancer, but they set out in the belief that they would find that some number of contributory causes had to operate in unison, like an orchestra playing a chord, for a cancer to begin.

Some of these causes would be in the environment (eg carcinogenic compounds or viruses). Some might be in the peasants' lifestyle and both of these would need to combine with some weaknesses in a particular person's internal defence system for the cancer to grow. The scientists believed that if they could find just some of the causes and remove them, then that might be enough.

Dr Yang, who was the senior scientist, an epidemiologist, recalled that when they arrived, because there was so much cancer, they had a fantastic welcome. They had to work out a plan to lead to prevention and cure, that was the first thing. But the task seemed dauntingly difficult.

During the first years of their experiment they could find no obvious causes. The area was free from industrial chemicals. There seemed nothing particularly special about the soil, save that it was low in a trace element – the metal molybdenum – and the well-water was slightly rich in nitrate and nitrite.

They looked for causes in the peasants' lifestyle. It seemed unexceptional. It was dominated by the need to grow enough food, to dry it and store it so they could survive the cold winter period. They grew cabbage, maize, wheat and turnips. The maize stalks were kept to burn; they were tied in bundles and stacked along the walls of the courtyards, forming a thick yellow hedge to each home. The corn cobs were hung in the sun to dry, so they would keep for making bread. They hung like plaits of yellow hair down the fronts of the white houses. The turnips and cabbages had to be dried, the turnips being grated and put out on the rooftops in the last of the autumn sun.

This lifestyle is similar to many parts of Northern China, but in this valley there had been an extreme shortage of water until a large irrigation scheme brought water only a decade ago. Ways of cooking that economised on water had become established, as had ways of preserving foods to endure not only one winter but through a drought and second winter too.

The scientists became suspicious of some aspects of this lifestyle: for example, the way that the peasants preserved persimmons (a soft fruit like a tomato) was to wrap it in a paste of sharp-pointed wheat husk. It was dried in the sun to a rock-hard cake – which would keep for ten years. The peasants used to eat the whole abrasive cake, and the scientists thought the repeated scratching of the food pipe was a cause.

Again, the way the peasants used to pickle vegetables came under suspicion. They made a kind of sauerkraut by rotting down cabbage leaves in stone jars. They used no salt or vinegar, just held the leaves under water, weighed down by a stone. After six weeks it would become an extremely acid pickle – grown over with a thick mould. It was a local delicacy.

Each group of homes used to have its own underground clay-lined cistern which they used to fill by hand when water was available. The scientists analysed this water and found that it had slightly more nitrate than is normal – but not at any level thought to be dangerous. However, the way they used it in cooking concentrated the chemicals. They used to steam their maize bread for hours, and the nitrite levels of the water in the bottom of the steamer was slightly high. But as that water was used to make soups, the nitrites in the food became mildly suspect.

People outside the valley had long said that the special cancer of Lin Xian was because they always ate their food too fast and too hot, that they were continually burning their oesophagus. That was one of the easiest things for the research team to investigate – and their findings showed that, although the people did bolt their food, it was no hotter there than elsewhere in China.

But they had hardly begun their research when the Cultural Revolution interrupted their work, in the mid-Sixties. The universities were closed, Western books burnt, the research in Lin Xian was stopped and the team dispersed into the vastness of China, to have their minds 'remoulded'. Only in the early Seventies was the work begun again.

Dr Li Bing, the Director of Research at the Cancer Research Institute of Peking, had the responsibility for reassembling the team. During the Cultural Revolution she had been assigned to the hospital laundry for two years, but the members of the team had kept in touch by letter.

One of the team in Lin Xian, Dr Liu, a pathologist working on the incidence of cancer of the gullet in chickens, said: 'We feared criticism. If you were working on experiments or in research, you "desired personal power and fame". The effect on my research was considerable. My work on the chickens stopped: I couldn't continue. You couldn't open a book without somebody criticising you. You couldn't look at a reference book in broad daylight! You read them on the sly at night. We did routine work every day, but no research.'

Dr Liu's work in chickens had begun during a survey when peasants had been asked if any of their families had difficulty in swallowing. One had said, 'No, but one of my chickens does.' That chicken when examined was found to have cancer of the gullet. And soon Dr Liu had established that the chicken cancer and the human cancer occurred together.

In 1970 Dr Liu could resume his work on chickens. He organised a survey of the 15,000 chickens in the most afflicted commune. He found that the chickens had the same incidence of cancer as the humans did. He got the barefoot doctors from the counties where the human cancer was very much less than that of Lin Xian to go looking for chickens with cancer. Some 40,000 chickens were examined, and the cancerous birds were sent to him. Some arrived on carts, some arrived with the postman, and some peasants walked miles to bring them. He found that where the human incidence was high, so it was in the chickens. Where it was low, it was low in the chickens too. The match between the incidence of human and chicken cancer was very close indeed.

This research raised questions. Was the cancer being passed from the chickens to the humans? Were the humans passing it to the chickens? Or were they both catching it independently from something in the environment? By a remarkable stroke of luck there had been a huge population migration that allowed the answer to be decided.

Some 50,000 people had had to move from a valley nearby because it was to be made into a reservoir. They suffered from the cancer. They were moved 300 miles to a district with little oesophageal cancer. They did not take their chickens with them, but were given new chickens when they got there. Dr Liu investigated this population.

Among the migrants' new chickens were twelve cases of cancer – a total contrast to the surrounding countryside, where the same stock of chickens were totally free of the disease. So it seemed certain that the chickens were getting it from the people. Most likely its origin was in the scraps and left-overs the peasants fed to them, so attention was focused on the Lin Xian diet.

During the Cultural Revolution a British scientist, Dr P. N. Magee, had published a report which the Chinese found extremely relevant. A certain group of compounds caused cancer of particular organs of experimental animals. Some of these compounds specifically went for the oesophagus. These compounds are called nitrosamines. They all have a similar structure – three branches forming a letter Y. One branch can be built from nitrite, and the other branches can be any amine fragments. Such fragments are often the products of decaying protein.

But there were no nitrosamines in the unpolluted rural environment. So scientists wondered if the nitrosamines were actually being made inside the peasants. Was it possible that in digesting local food the stomach could be manufacturing these lethal carcinogenic chemicals?

To find out, an experiment was done on five pigs waiting to be butchered at the main slaughterhouse in Lin Xian. Small amounts of nitrite and amine fragments (made from local wheat) were added to the pigs' food, and the pigs were allowed to digest their spiked meal for an hour. As soon as each pig was butchered, its stomach was given intact to a scientist, who rushed it on his bicycle to be analysed. In the laboratory it was proved that the chemical *had* linked to become nitrosamines. So the hunt began for the fragments in the human diet from which it was possible that the nitrosamines were being made. Dr Li and the scientists from Peking started to look for the nitrite ingredient. She began by measuring the nitrite levels in the peasants. She analysed the urine of twenty-seven women, and found that they carried in their bodies a great deal of nitrite. From the urine she estimated their vitamin levels. Their vitamin C level turned out to be extremely low – so she gave the women extra vitamin C for a week and measured nitrite levels again. They had dropped to almost one third. It seemed to the Chinese that lack of vitamin C interfered with the body's natural defence against nitrite. So two unrelated facts now fell into a pattern.

The research team had already found the local soil was low in the trace element, molybdenum, and from reading Western research they could now see the significance of that. Low molybdenum was seriously affecting, not the humans, but the plants. Without enough molybdenum, plants concentrate nitrite in their leaves – and they make less vitamin C. So the people were doubly at risk from nitrite. It was concentrated in their vegetables – and without enough vitamin C their bodies natural defence systems couldn't protect them from it.

So it became clear where one part of the nitrosamine molecule came from. Where did the rest – the amines – come from, the fragments that come from decaying protein? Moulds grow very easily in the valley: almost anything gets a mould on it after being stored for a few weeks. The scientists now became interested in the moulds the peasants ate as part of their diet.

The locals made a steamed bread from corn flour; and to conserve fuel and water they made enough at one time to last them for three weeks. The bread started to go mouldy after a few days, but the peasants seemed to like that, just as some people in the West like the mould in blue cheese. When samples of the bread were allowed to go mouldy in the laboratory, it was found that in hundreds of cases the results were quite harmless. But a few fungi created the levels of amine fragments in the bread to increase rapidly. One fungus, F.moniliforum, was especially powerful in this respect: it caused a seventeenfold increase in two days. So they believed they had uncovered the source of the second half of the nitrosamine. It was the action of fungus on food.

Then they discovered something unexpected – a result which may have significance outside Lin Xian. Not only did laboratory rats eating mouldy bread with added nitrite get cancer: for a few moulds, the control rats on mouldy bread alone got cancer too. The moulds could create the nitrite part of the nitrosamine themselves. Since then the Chinese have found that some moulds can make nitrosamines directly, and are possibly pro-

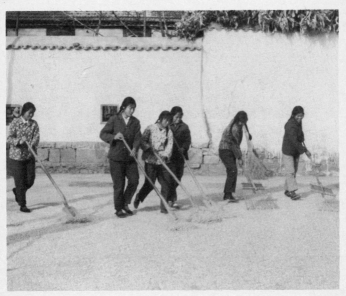

Since 1975 corn has been dried to prevent fungus growing on it during storage.

ducing their own cancer-causing agents, as yet unidentified. In order to find which moulds are dangerous the scientists have started growing pure strains of the local fungi. But the work will take years, for there are 10,000 local fungi – and each experiment involves waiting two years to see whether the rats will develop a cancer.

By 1974, the research team felt that if peasants avoided all the factors they had come to suspect, then cancer of the oesophagus would be eradicated in the Lin Xian valley. The campaign against this cancer is mobilising the 70,000 villagers at the worst affected end of the valley. In each village the barefoot doctor is responsible for constant propaganda, to remind them continuously only to drink the purified piped water which has had nitrate and nitrite removed, to eat fresh vegetables, and not to make the persimmon cakes or the pickled vegetables that the locals like so much. And, particularly, *not* to eat mouldy food.

To prevent mould growing in stored foods, large drying areas have been constructed – barns built on waterproof platforms. To overcome the lack of molybdenum in the soil, a small amount of this element is added to the seeds before they are planted – ammonium molybdate is dissolved in water, and the seeds soaked with it. As a result, in the wheat and maize grown now, there is forty per cent less nitrite, and in the vegetables there is twenty-five per cent more vitamin C. The pace of the work has been very fast. Work could only begin on the fungus and nitrosamines in 1970 – and yet by 1974 the anti-cancer campaign had begun.

As it takes years for a cancer to develop, Dr Yang thinks it will be a long time before we can tell if the new regime stops the cancer? 'After a period of time the cancer rate might drop: it may take ten years. If it drops, we'll know our suspicions are correct. If the rate doesn't drop, we were wrong. It's a tough job to change a people's way of life. But we've confidence that *in time* we'll have some clear-cut answers.'

During the decade over which the preventive measures have been developed the people had to be treated. The Lin Xian hospitals were coping with a steady stream of cases, and what they were able to do was a major operation to remove the cancer, much as would be done in the West.

Most of the cancers were advanced and the patient near death, because by the time a patient feels the first symptoms, the cancer is typically well developed: it was said that if you first felt it in springtime you would not survive the winter. For what begins as

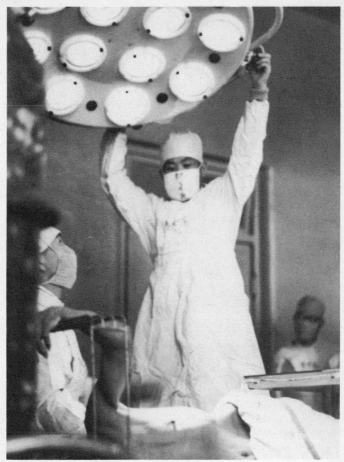

Operation on an old lady for suspected cancer of the oesophagus.

a mild sensation, roughly like a fragment of lettuce leaf that you can't swallow, becomes within ten months a total blockage.

Professor Shen is an eminent pathologist who chose early in his career to live in this remote valley. He decided to look for some way of finding the cancer before the symptoms developed – while it was smaller and more curable – and even hoped to find a pre-malignant stage at which the progress to cancer might be halted or even turned back.

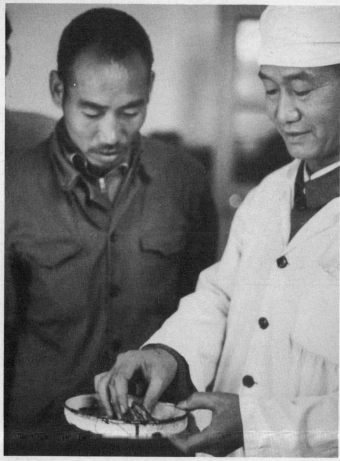

The surgeon shows the patient's son the cancerous growth he has removed.

He developed a way of making huge slides – almost as big as bacon rashers – from the hundreds of oesophageal specimens that were being removed by the surgeons. As he explored the differences between the normal tissue and the invading edge of the cancer he found there was a non-serious pre-malignant state, in which the wall of the oesophagus thickens, but the over-growth is not out of control – much as the cells in a wart don't multiply and invade the tissue. He found this condition, called hyperplasia, could turn to cancer and the cancer could grow unfelt for several years. Shen's next move was to devise a simple test with which to detect this symptomless cancer.

This he achieved in 1958 when he put on the end of a thin plastic pipe a small balloon contained in a fine mesh bag. While deflated, the balloon was swallowed all the way down into the patient's stomach. Then he inflated the balloon (to about the size of a tomato) and as he pulled it up, the mesh took a scraping of the oesophagus. From the scraping Shen could tell if the person was normal, if he had hyperplasia, or if a cancer had begun. Between 1958-62 he tried it on numerous people till he became confident he could detect a cancer with accuracy.

In 1964 this knowledge was put to the test. Shen was convinced by his tests that a peasant had a cancer, but the surgeon said, 'I can't feel anything, the man has no symptoms, and X-rays shows nothing, so how can I operate on the basis of your evidence, which I don't believe in.' Shens reply was, 'How can you let a cancer develop when I know it is there – and I guarantee it's there.' The surgeon refused. Shen repeated the balloon test, and again demonstrated the cancer cells. The argument went on for hours until in a mixture of angry emphasis and genuine challenge, Shen said, 'If you don't find a cancer when you operate, then he can have my oesophagus.' The surgeon started the operation and couldn't find a cancer. He called Shen, who took a sample from the man on the table and found a small cancer. It was less than 1 cm across, but it was definite. The surgeon completed the operation, and after this surgeons generally accepted Shen's test.

The story spread far, and with it the popularity of Shen's balloon test – even though it's quite painful, and leaves a powerful sore throat. By 1970 the barefoot doctors had been shown how to do the test and a survey was done of *everyone's* oesophagus in the valley – amounting to 70,000 people. There was another mass survey in 1978. From these surveys a surprising picture emerged of the growth of the cancer: half the population at any one time had mild thickening of the oesophagus or hyperplasia. It seemed that people repeatedly switched between this condition and normality. About twelve per cent of those who had developed the mild form went on to the severe thickening; and once that had developed over one third of these people regressed to normal again. In about one sixth of these people the severe thickening developed into cancer. This step was irreversible, but it took a long time, for half of the peasants took longer than twelve years to go from severe hyperplasia to cancer.

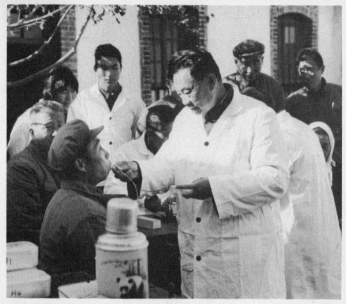

Dr Shen, inventor of the balloon tests, carrying out a routine village screening programme.

Plainly, if they could halt the progress from hyperplasia to cancer, they would have achieved control of the disease. They are trying to achieve that control with drugs. One drug that is being used very widely is *Kongai i San* (literally translated, it means 'fight cancer drug no. 3'). It is made in a local factory from a brew of chopped herbs, and is indeed one of the drugs of traditional Chinese medicine, although its conventional use is to 'draw out high temperature', and the traditional doctors of China don't know of its anti-cancer properties.

There are many peasants on these drugs whose hyperplasia has been cured, and many whose hyperplasia has not progressed to cancer for periods of up to sixteen years. Whether these patients would have stayed well without this treatment is not known. It's only recently that the comparative clinical trials have begun. In a one-year experiment, begun in 1977, it was found that, in a sample of 215 people who had no treatment, thirty per cent returned to normal in that year, whereas in seventy-two cases on *Kongai i San*, seventy-five per cent returned to normal.

Kongai i San is just one of the thousands of medicines used in

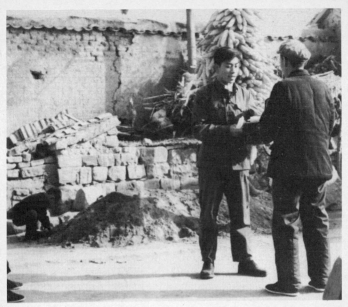

A barefoot doctor gives a herbal remedy to a man who has suffered from hyperplasia for 16 years.

traditional Chinese medicine, a rich heritage of drugs that is now being worked through and tested systematically for their anti-cancer properties. Such untested drugs cannot, obviously, be given to people with severe hyperplasia: when the Chinese have a belief in *Kongai i San* they can hardly give a person on the verge of cancer another drug which may well be useless. So they have developed two screening tests. Firstly, they have found that beansprouts react to known anti-cancer drugs much as tumours do, that drugs known to be effective against cancer stop them growing, ineffective ones don't. So row upon row of germinating beansprouts are laid out, various herbal extracts are put into their dishes, and the beans are grown for three days. Those drugs which stunt the plants' growth are chosen for more detailed assessment. The importance of the 'beansprout' screening is that it's something the barefoot doctors can set up in their particular villages.

Secondly, in contrast to the rudimentary bean test one of the virologists, Dr Ge Ming, has developed a most sophisticated screening technique. He has successfully kept alive cancer cells that he took from the cancer of a woman who died in 1973. (The culture is called Cell line 109, because he failed in the previous 108 attempts.) It is thus on live human cancer cells that the traditional drugs are being assessed. The drug is put in with the cancer cells, and Dr Ge Ming can tell within days if it attacks them. He has found so far at least ten herbs and roots that are extremely active, but he is cautious about making claims. He says that they haven't been tried on humans yet. He won't publish anything until the clinical trials are held. But he's excited by the anti-cancer drugs he's finding.

At the centre of the Lin Xian valley is the county hospital. A notification of every case of cancer in the valley goes into the records held there. There is a similar organisation in every province of China – each barefoot doctor, notifies the registry in his district of each case of cancer, its diagnosis, and how the patient fares. The information from all the registries is compiled and analysed at the Peking Cancer Institution, and thus a total picture of the cancer problem in China is built up. The figures are used to update maps – one for each type of cancer.

And each map reveals surprising patterns – clues for new directions of research. For example, the most recent pattern for male lung cancer shows that it is concentrated in the industrial parts of the country. But it also shows an isolated region where lung cancer is common in a rural district of Canton. The maps for cancer of the back of the nose show that the disease is concentrated in the southern part of China. The map for liver cancer shows it to be concentrated along the coast, especially around Shanghai. The pattern for liver cancer generally is different from the pattern of liver cancer among women. Each map poses questions and they suggest new areas to explore.

The Chinese approach is characterised by close contact between the scientist and the people. And the teams are involved simultaneously in both treatment and research.

They focus on big, single problems, and their goal is not so much to understand the detail as to arrive at a basis for practical action. With little equipment, they have had to use the co-operation of a large disciplined population as their primary tool.

Their approach to cancer is different from ours. They have not concentrated on high technology laboratories. They are not looking for the hidden key to cancer inside the cell. They are not searching for the molecular mechanisms at the critical moment when a cell turns into a cancer. Their way has been different. In many ways it is a complementary approach to ours. It is good that, as their isolation is ending, we in the West can benefit from their work, just as they have benefited from ours.

The Contributors

SIMON CAMPBELL-JONES has been a producer since 1967, making mostly science programmes for BBC-TV and WGBH Boston. He was Editor of *Horizon* from 1976–81.

ROBIN BRIGHTWELL joined the BBC as a graduate with qualifications in agriculture and biochemistry. He has produced several *Horizon* films, as well as BBC1 documentaries, on subjects such as The Pill, Bone-Marrow transplants, Deep-Sea Diving and Tunnelling. He was series producer on *The Human Brain*, and co-authored the book of the series with Dick Gilling.

DOMINIC FLESSATI taught biology before joining the BBC, where he worked in External Services and the *Radio Times* before becoming a television producer. As producer he worked on *Tomorrow's World*, on the *Controversy* series from the Royal Institution, and on *The Secret War*. His many *Horizons* include 'What Time is your Body?', 'Dragnet for Diabetes' and 'The Mondragon Experiment'.

MARTIN FREETH, after a degree in Philosophy and Politics, studied film and television at the Royal College of Art, and worked as a film editor before joining the Science and Features department of BBC television in 1971. His work includes *The Burke Special*, major Science Specials such as *Einstein's Universe*, and *Horizons* on 'The Spike' (epilepsy), 'The Mind's Eye' (the visual system) and 'Darwin's Dream'. He recently finished directing a drama-documentary about Sir Cyril Burt.

DICK GILLING is a graduate in English Literature who has written and produced more than fifty science programmes. They include many for *Horizon* as well as episodes of *The Ascent of Man*, *The Age of Uncertainty* and *Human Brain*.

EDWARD GOLDWYN is married with three daughters. After reading physics joined the BBC Schools department in 1962 and then moved to Further Education, to the Open University and to help set up the Community Programme Unit. Since joining *Horizon* in 1975 he has made sixteen films for the series and received nine awards.

VIVIENNE KING's first job in the BBC was with the newly-established Open University. In 1973 she moved to the Science and Features Department, where she has produced numerous *Horizons* ('Mr Ludwig's Tropical Dreamland', 'Voices from Silent Hands') as well as two series of *Medical Express*.

Picture Credits

Dr El-Alamy, Center for Field and Applied Research, Egyptian Ministry of Health p. 148; American Legion, Pennsylvania 112; Associated Press 115; Committee for Community Relations, Cape Town 100; Communicable Diseases Centre, Colindale 128; Dr Susanne Isaacs Elmhirst 10; Glasgow District Libraries 26; C. Goldwyn 156, 161, 163, 164, 166, 167; E. Goldwyn 102; R. Goldwyn 145; International General Electric Co. of New York Ltd 45; Lehtikuva Oy 14; Dr D. J. McLaren, Division of Parasitology, NIMR 142; MRC Dunn Nutrition Unit, Cambridge 30; MRC Reproductive Biology Unit, Edinburgh 96; Philadelphia Inquirer (photo William F. Steinmetz) 113; Royal College of Surgeons 44; Dr M. J. Stock 38; US Center for Disease Control 121, 122, 123, 125; Wellcome Foundation 141; Mrs Went 98; WHO 140, 150.